"People involved in therapeutic and community gardens will find this book an invaluable guide to creating gardens and groups that offer maximum benefit to everyone involved. Both rookie and expert gardeners will see their vocation in a fascinating new light. For every reader, gardener or not, this book offers a wealth of profoundly thought-provoking ideas about what it means to be well and live well."

Fiona Thackeray,
Head of Operations & Development, **Trellis Scotland**

"*The Garden Cure* is the book many community gardeners and anyone interested in gardening and good mental health have been waiting for ... moving, insightful ... Packed with real life stories and insights from the author's decades of experience working in the field ... this book will be an invaluable read for anyone working alongside others in a garden setting ...I will refer to it for many years to come."

Louisa Evans, Scotland Development Worker,
Social Farms and Gardens

"Jan Cameron has distilled more than forty years of experience of working with groups in gardens and outdoors into a book full of wisdom and very sound advice ... illustrated in a thoughtful way that will assist people with ... literacy problems. [The book is] as useful and as accessible to those who have mental health problems themselves as it is to those

Reforesting Scotland Journal

T0284697

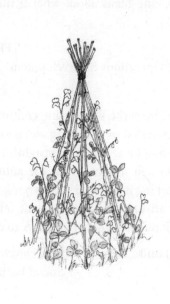

THE GARDEN CURE

Cultivating our well-being and growth

Jan Cameron

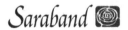

Published by Saraband
Digital World Centre, 1 Lowry Plaza,
The Quays, Salford, M50 3UB
www.saraband.net

ISBN: 9781912235872
ebook: 9781912235995

1 2 3 4 5 6 7 8 9 10

Printed and bound in Great Britain by Clays Ltd, Elcograf S.p.A.

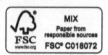

MIX
Paper from
responsible sources
FSC® C018072

CONTENTS

PREFACE

This book is intended for anyone with an interest in gardens and the ways in which they help us to understand ourselves and make us feel better about what happens in our lives. I hope it will be every bit as relevant to the general public as it is to professionals working in the broad fields of health and well-being, horticulture and therapy.

In the same way that first aid courses have been rolled out to every sector in our society to raise awareness of simple tools to help people manage medical situations, so too should mental health first aid and tools for well-being be available to the general public. This might help to stem the epidemic of poor mental health that our society is experiencing. I know of no better place to start than in the garden.

While much of my working life has been spent in therapeutic gardens designed for people experiencing mental health problems, both adults and children, for the last seven years I have been very involved with community gardens, and the lessons learnt in the first context have been just as relevant in the second.

Recent years have seen a huge increase in the demand for community gardens and allotments all over the country and internationally. In particular, the benefits that gardening can have for personal well-being have generated a huge upsurge of interest in the topic.

I hope this book will be of use to anyone who wants to engage in community gardening – and many people do. The recollections, stories and tools described should also be helpful to anyone who is experiencing distress, or supporting someone else in their distress, whatever their interests.

All of the stories are anonymised and, although they may seem specific to an individual, they are most often a compilation of many different stories and experiences. Any association with a particular name is entirely coincidental. For the ease of the reader, I usually refer simply to 'the garden' whereas in fact the stories come from many different gardens. While all of our journeys are different, our common humanity throws up many similarities in the ways we perceive and respond to life's challenges.

PART ONE

IN THE GARDEN

GROWING WELL IN GARDENS

This is a story of gardens and how people can grow well in them. There is something in the whole metaphor of gardening that helps us to understand the way we ourselves grow and thrive and blossom. You see, it starts right away in the language we use to describe our well-being. We 'languish' or we 'flourish'. We talk of people, especially children, 'blossoming', and pregnant women are 'blooming'. We speak of our work 'bearing fruit', young girls 'in the flower of their youth'. Elderly people are sometimes described as 'withered'. When we look at the story of the garden, it is the story of ourselves. We are intricately intertwined.

Why do we create these places? Is it to provide safety and protection for plants that would otherwise fail? Is it an attempt to make a safe place for ourselves to retreat to? What is it about them that brings us such pleasure? Is there an innate connection and bounty? The studies made of the 'green effect' are numerous and convincing, from Edward Wilson's *Biophilia*[1] and *Shin Rin-Yoku*[2] (Japanese tree bathing) to the discovery of beneficial bacteria in the soil having an effect similar to Prozac in alleviating depression[3]. This study, however, is a story based on a lifetime's experience rather than scientific study, although several studies will be alluded to.

The purpose of this book, and my desire in writing it, is to capture some of what I and many others have learnt – and indeed discovered daily – through the experiences of working over decades in therapeutic and community gardens. It is noteworthy how what works for plants replicates closely the way we grow and develop as humans. We will explore the parallels between the phases of work in the garden and how they mirror human needs.

> *"What is true about a healthy mind and body is true in creating a healthy garden."*
>
> Monty Don[4]

I've been lucky to work in remarkable places with remarkable people throughout my career. At a young age, just eighteen years old, a chance decision undoubtedly changed the course of my life and work. After what would have been described then as a working-class upbringing in Edinburgh, instead of taking up a university place I decided to volunteer as a Community Service Volunteer (CSV)[5] and was sent to a hostel for pregnant homeless women, mostly very young girls, in London. The principles there were of dignity, respect and unfailing kindness. This served to steer my path towards an interest in the politics of poverty and distress and to learn about the means to alleviate those conditions.

I went on to work in a grim psycho-geriatric ward in a Glasgow hospital. Then, after a three-year course in community education, I spent ten years working as the gardener in the walled garden of a pioneering residential school for emotionally distressed young boys. It was here that I first discovered the power of the garden to influence a fragile state of being for the better. I was privileged to learn more about the healing powers of compassion and humane and clever inventiveness. Twenty-five years followed, working in therapeutic gardens for adults experiencing mental health problems, gaining new insights every day, even and especially on the worst days. I have spent the last seven years working in community gardens in the Scottish Borders and I am loving every minute of it.

COMMUNITY GARDENING

Community gardens come in all sorts of different shapes and sizes. Some can be several acres, others can be the size of a typical council house back garden. Some are managed as a part of a much bigger mental health, environmental or social organisation; some are national, some are small, individual and local. They can also vary in management styles. As part of a big organisation, some gardens have a paid staff team and have to adhere to company rules and guidelines, while others are managed by boards of trustees or committee and may have a very small staff team or a single worker. Then there are those that have no structure at all and are run democratically or even anarchically by a small group of unpaid individuals with no budget. They all involve volunteers and as such share a great deal of common experience. I have worked in all kinds of these settings and it is this commonality I would like to describe.

In these pages, I have distilled some of what I have observed and learnt along the way about the close interaction between horticulture and better mental health.

The garden itself is a wonderful metaphor for health. Organics in horticulture is all about creating the conditions for health rather than treating the symptoms of disease. It is easy to see the parallels with the human condition. In horticultural terms when we try to create a healthy growing environment, we look at good nutrition and regular watering specific to each plant's needs. We need good hygiene routines, to prune out unproductive growth and concentrate energy on the healthy branches, to keep on top of the weeds, to encourage fresh air, with time to rest and room to grow and unfold safely. Does this ring any bells?

Here is just one story that illustrates how powerfully this can work. We will explore many such examples throughout the course of the book. (As mentioned before, every story and example in this book is drawn from the real experiences of different people, but I have distilled common elements of these into a single story – and I have always anonymised them.)

One morning Josh came into the garden and his body language was the picture of dejection. He wore a baseball hat firmly pulled over his face. His shoulders were slumped, his back was rounded and his eyes were downcast. He was carefully trying to avoid catching anyone's eye or engaging with anyone. His body language was saying very clearly: "I am feeling very fragile and afraid. Please don't come near me." When I watched him put his boots on I could see he was trembling. We knew from experience that this was not a good time to try and talk to him about why he was feeling low, so we assigned him a task in the garden as usual. His job for the day was to tie back the branches of the apple trees on the south-facing wall. Luckily, it was a warm sunny day.

Two hours later when I went to check on him he was fully engaged in the task. He was standing with the sun on his back, which was easing all his muscles, he had his arms outstretched on either side in order to reach the bits of the tree he had to tie up. His back had straightened, his chest had opened, his head had come up, he was breathing deeply and he was talking to the person standing next to him – because he had to, so that they could put the ties up together. It was like a lesson in several alternative therapies – yoga, Alexander Technique, tai chi, mindfulness, massage and talking therapies all rolled into one – AND the tree got supported and we got apples!

It's that subtle combination of things that opens people up and helps them to talk and feel more at ease.

I refer frequently to four gardens that were also mental health services. The lessons learnt there apply just as readily to community gardens, allotment groups and indeed creative groups of many different kinds. I worked in these gardens for more than thirty-five years, and they are dear to my heart. Together, we cultivated them into healthy, thriving organic havens for people recovering from mental health problems – and indeed, as the adult ones were open to the public, they provided an oasis for anyone who came into contact with them. My hope is that these accumulated experiences may be of interest and use to you and those whom you may meet or work with, just as all gardens and all people can grow and flourish with a little attention and shared knowledge.

Throughout the book, I will refer to people attending these gardens as volunteers (with the exception of the children's unit), and the gardens as therapeutic gardens as opposed to community gardens. By volunteers, I mean people who have made a personal choice to come to work in the garden without payment, with the hope of finding a safe space, some peace from their distress, and inspiration: places that neither look nor feel like a medical setting, but a place of work.

The gardens and the work that happened within them were the result of very dedicated and skilled teams of people who were willing to give their best. They were creative, curious, honest, and a privilege to know and work with.

I loved going to work and looked forward to every day. Even the difficult parts, like when someone was telling me about something awful that had happened to them, gave me the privilege of being trusted with something very special – despite it being about stressful and often deeply sad situations. I was always inspired by the courage that people showed. The world feels a better place to me with the knowledge that there are places where people feel safe enough to open up and share and support each other and believe in a future for themselves.

The beauty of working with people in a garden is that it is most definitely a place of work with a clear 'firmly rooted' agenda of 'creating growth' for the future. (As you may have realised by now, it is also a place that yields metaphors!) We, and others, benefit from it, but it is not about us. It's a chance to have a break from our own problems and dilemmas and to get involved, immersed, absorbed in a completely different universe: the world of plants, the weather, nature and its many creatures. It's both hard work and restful at the same time. After a day in the garden you feel pleasantly tired, rather than worn out. Gradually, your body becomes fitter and your mind begins to relax.

WHAT KIND OF PEOPLE COME HERE?

If I had a pound for every member of the public who came to visit a therapeutic garden and asked me this question in the last twenty-five years, I would be dining out every week. What kind of people come here? Their implication seemed to be that it couldn't possibly be the kind of people they knew, and certainly not themselves. My usual response would be, "People like you and me. There is no special kind of person who comes here. We have professional people, craftsmen, teachers, doctors, plumbers, chefs, artists, manual workers, and some people who have never had paid work. We have visitors from a whole range of educational achievements, all ethnicities, religious backgrounds, and physical abilities".

As one person in the garden noted, she had never worked with such a diverse group of people in her life. Usually we spend most of our lives with people in the same profession – whether engineers, architects, teachers, social workers or other occupations – or their client group, customers and suppliers. The mix in the garden makes for a different kind of learning experience in itself.

While out walking recently, I was thinking about this and suddenly realised that there was in fact a common denominator. People come to a therapeutic garden because they want their lives to be different. They have that very particular kind of courage that it takes to walk through the gates of a strange place and meet someone like me – someone they don't know. Moreover, they have the courage to admit that their lives are not going the way they want them to, and that perhaps they need help to change things. I still don't know after all these years whether I would have the courage to do that myself.

The people I worked with taught me a language to describe their emotional inner journey and their recovery experience, especially when it followed a lifetime of abuse or trauma. They laid an easier path for someone who would come after them, and this helped me to work more effectively with the next person. Although we never go down the same recovery path twice, the person before often provided a gate or a stepping stone into the next person's story, aiding a better understanding. Indeed, as everyone wore the same clothing – steel toe-capped boots and work jeans – people visiting the garden were often not aware of whether they were talking to a member of staff or a volunteer.

This book is a tribute to all those brave people and everything they were able to teach, however painful that process was for them. Hopefully many of them feel that by sharing their stories they've opened up possibilities for others to be helped, and that some good will have come out of their distress.

I have seen over and over how people's lives can be transformed – put back together and changed for the better – by the richly healing rhythms of growing together in a garden.

If I contributed in any way to make the gardens I worked in better places for anyone to be in, then I feel grateful to have had that opportunity.

THE MAGIC OF A WALLED GARDEN

The majority of my working life has been spent in walled gardens, which all dated from the late eighteenth or early nineteenth century. A walled garden is not a passing whim. It's built to last for centuries. There is something very reassuring about being in a space that has been dedicated to gardening over a long period of time.

Each of these gardens had to be restored from a sadly neglected state. Visitors and volunteers would often comment on the sense of sanctuary, even of enchantment, in these beautiful spaces. Beauty and magic were created every day by the people who worked there.

The basic layout of the gardens tends to be similar in design. Here's what a typical one might look and feel like.

The garden is built on a slight slope, south facing and about the size of a couple of football pitches, with a river running along just behind the bottom wall. The walls and the whole garden are cleverly designed to keep a flow of warmer air travelling through, to protect the early blossom and help ripen the fruit of the trees trained against the top, south-facing wall.

As you walk along the path towards the walled garden, the gate beckons to you, and when you pass through it's as if you've stepped into another world. A walled garden is almost always a fair distance from any modern road, and so there is no traffic noise. It is surrounded by mature woodland, which adds to the special kind of hush, broken only by the birds singing, the sound of the river, and the occasional voices drifting up from one of the beds where people work quietly away, and maybe the hum of a lawnmower somewhere nearby.

Once inside the garden you will find that it is divided into a series of 'rooms' – different and distinct spaces – and pathways with hedges giving only tantalising glimpses of what lies behind them, of what comes next. The paths will invite you to walk round, and as you do you will come across herbaceous flowerbeds with their riot of colours, leafy arbours and rose beds. You will find quiet places to sit and contemplate, herb beds quite formally laid out, often in the shape of a wheel, and shrub borders along the north facing wall. In the heart of the garden there is likely to be a pond somewhere; ponds look beautiful and frogs and toads are great for keeping slugs at bay. The sound of water adds a real sense of tranquillity to the garden and helps to create the calming atmosphere of this special place.

There will be vegetable beds: potatoes, cabbages, beetroot and parsnips, onions and leeks, tall canes supporting peas and beans. People will be working in all these beds at their own pace, to keep on top of the weeds and care for the crop. As you move up the garden to the south-facing wall there are likely to be currant bushes, raspberries and gooseberries all growing under cages of netting to keep the birds from stealing them. Strawberries will have straw tucked under them to keep them clean and fresh. Against the wall there will be apple, pear, plum and fig trees basking in the warmth radiated by the wall itself, which holds the heat of the sun.

The hedges that surround each area will be home to lots of wildlife: birds, mice, voles and insects. These hedges will take it in turn to flower and fruit and provide an ever-changing backdrop to these garden 'rooms'. Often at the corners there will be trees that give shade and colour, and roosting spots for the birds you need to help control the insects – many of which also play an important role – and to bring more shade, colour and delight. There will surely be lovingly filled bird feeders hanging from the trees, regularly raided by cheerful and cheeky squirrels.

Last but most definitely not least will be the composting area. This will have compost heaps, leaf mould heaps, wood piles, stone piles and general recycling. Every year this corner sees the magical transformation of garden waste into rich, fertile compost. I always judge a garden by its composting!

It is this environment – rich in history; peaceful but dynamic; ever-evolving yet providing a still, calming centre; full of interest; and beautiful on so many different levels – which provides the therapeutic setting for the work and ideas which we will explore over the course of this book.

If I do my job right, then the world will be a little bit more beautiful and people will be a little bit happier. What more could anybody wish from their life?

James Alexander-Sinclair[6]

KEY POINTS

- A garden is a place of work with an agenda firmly rooted in the future.

- People can work together without having to share or dwell on their past.

- Working in the garden gives people a chance to take some 'time off' from their anxieties.

CHAPTER I

DISCOVERING THE GARDEN

There is a moment of excitement when you enter a new garden for the first time. It's like the beginning of a love affair. You look forward to finding out all that is growing there, knowing that every day will bring a fresh wonder from the earth.

If your first visit is in the chilly depths of winter, it can look like an empty landscape with little going on. It can be tempting at this stage to rush in with lots of enthusiasm and great plans and start digging it over and laying out new beds, paying no heed to what might lie underneath.

However, if you are prepared to wait and get to know your garden slowly as the ground thaws each day, it will choose to disclose new things; these will burst through and come to flower, and you will gradually come to understand it. You will learn how the trees look when they are in full leaf, where the shadows fall in midsummer, and where the sunny spots are. You should do little more than careful weeding, feeding and support in that first year or you may unwittingly damage the unseen growth below the ground. You may choose to sow a few annuals (plants with a life cycle of one year only) in bare patches, tilling the soil very lightly so as to do no harm, and simply watch and wait to see what comes. You might study the weeds as they can tell you a lot about the kind of soil you have.

MAKING THE RELATIONSHIP

New people coming into a busy garden can appear reserved at first, and it can be hard to see what problems they're dealing with. As a health worker/garden leader it is important that you approach each new relationship with the same excitement and wonder you would a new garden.

As I once wrote in an article for the Scottish Recovery Network: "If someone comes through the door today and they are brand new to me I need to be brand new for them. I need to be really keen to meet that person and find out who they are and what they like and don't like, what they want and don't want, in a way that needs to be fresh and open. I need to be excited and I need to want to do it."

Jack came to the garden after a long period in a psychiatric hospital, following a breakdown caused by abuse in his childhood. Thoughts and memories that he had been managing to suppress most of his life had started to surface, filling him with dread and hopelessness. He appeared to be very depressed. He was quiet, in fact he could barely speak, and engaging with others seemed like torture for him. At this point I had no idea what his story was, and I didn't know much about his background. Later I found out that he was actually a singing teacher, yet he had literally lost his voice.

It would have been easy to rush in with lots of chatter and 'helpful' advice with useful tips for dealing with depression, etc. It is really hard to sit quietly with that amount of distress.

However, as I am sure you know from your own hard times, what people need most in that moment is for you to find a way of quietly being there without being too intrusive, until they begin to feel safe. A garden is the perfect setting to provide quiet places where you can work companionably and purposefully alongside someone.

People can then begin to tell their story, often not verbally. Janice showed feelings of isolation in the way she spent most of her time locked in her bedsit, only going out when she absolutely had to, often doing her shopping late at night when the store was quiet. But at that time, of course, the city streets could be more dangerous. Her lack of trust in others, and more poignantly in herself, was evident in the way she went off to have lunch alone every day instead of joining in the small groups of other volunteers. She also found it very difficult to work in a group and to attend the site meeting (a weekly meeting for everyone in the garden). As time passed and she began to feel safer, she gradually managed to do all of these things.

Jack always said he didn't do talking or crying even though he often seemed very distressed in the garden. I had respected this for several years thinking he just didn't want to tell his story. I was talking to some students one day about trauma and suddenly mid-speech it hit me that he had been telling me his story all along. He always wore short-sleeved T-shirts and his arms were covered in scars from self-harming. (This wasn't unusual in itself). He made no attempt to cover them up; if anything, quite the opposite, he made them very visible. I suddenly saw with awful clarity that he had been showing me the pain he was in all along. When I went back out to the garden, I said I was sorry he had suffered so much, and suddenly we were talking and crying, and he began the slow process of putting his story into words and hopefully beginning to heal.

I have found that people's behaviour, no matter how strange it might seem, always starts to make sense when you begin to understand their story. As you start to understand someone's story and what is going on for them you can begin to offer some seeds of helpful ideas that might take root when the conditions are right. You might have to do a lot of research and studying to find the right seeds. Or indeed just listen and bear witness to their narrative.

Remember that the conditions have to be right for seeds to germinate, and some seeds lie dormant for a long time before they eventually sprout. This will be happening on many levels with lots of different people, including yourself.

WORKING TOGETHER IN A GARDEN
CHANGES EVERYONE

Working together to produce something beautiful and productive is in itself a wonderful form of therapy. Working alongside others in a garden on something bigger and other than yourself, is, in the words of the Canadian social psychologist Corey Keyes[7], in the realms of 'living life to the full'.

LANGUISHING TO FLOURISHING

Keyes describes the continuum we all exist on as 'from languishing to flourishing'. There is an ocean of difference between flourishing and being merely symptom free or in control of symptoms.

Louise came into mental health services as someone diagnosed with schizophrenia and hearing voices. When she first started at the garden, she was severely overweight (a common side effect of some psychiatric medications) and found it difficult to work physically or to concentrate for any length of time. Since starting her medication, she was free from hearing voices and was no longer having psychotic episodes. She had been discharged from hospital care, yet she still struggled because she had no energy, and her weight and poor concentration meant she could not do the things she wanted to. She was really keen to move out of services and into work, and she never missed a day in the garden.

Thinking we might be able to support her ambitions to be more active and eventually find employment, we arranged a meeting with her psychiatrist to see if we could work out a solution between us.

Both Louise and her fellow gardeners explained how challenging it was for her to take part in the work, despite her determination. She found it difficult to focus on any task. Her weight gain made physical jobs very tiring for her. Her medical team thought Louise was doing very well indeed. Most of the patients who were on a similar dosage even found it difficult to get out of bed. Her efforts were the equivalent of you or me trying to function having drunk a bottle of whisky.

The meeting didn't do much good for Louise at that point, but it did make us realise how much effort she had been making and so it helped to adjust our attitudes and responses.

With Louise we needed that crucial extra piece of information to understand her behaviour, just as in a garden. If, for example, you want to grow blueberries, you need to know that they need an acidic soil in order to flourish. When encountering people, plants or gardens for the first time, discovery and an understanding of the right support and best conditions for growth can take many different forms.

KEY POINTS

Discovering the garden

- Approach every encounter with curiosity and wonder, as if setting out on an exciting journey.

- Try to still yourself to listen and observe quietly, without rushing in with lots of chatter and advice.

- People need to be allowed time until they feel safe enough to tell their story. Often, they will tell it in non-verbal ways.

- Once you understand someone's story, their behaviour will start to make sense.

- Working together in partnership changes everyone.

CHAPTER 2

PREPARING THE GROWING ENVIRONMENT

There are many decisions to be made when you prepare a new garden. Some are matters of principles or ethics, whilst others are purely practical:

- Are you going to use chemicals or be organic?

- Are you going to grow fruit and vegetables or only decorative plants, or a mixture?

- Are you a private garden or open to the public?

- Are you aiming for a formal layout or a cottage garden effect?

- Where are you going to put the greenhouse or polytunnel?

- Who is going to work in the garden?

- Do you want to start a mood board – a collection of pictures of styles, colours and shapes that inspire you?

There are all kinds of things you might have to consider, such as whether to move a whole lot of debris from the area, build fences or walls to protect it, look at old plans to find water courses and the routes of previous paths, or take down any old or diseased trees that might be a hazard. If the garden is going to be open to the public, you must think about access and publicity.

Planning of this kind will give you a start. However, in the well-known words of Robert Burns, 'the best laid plans of mice and men gang aft agley': things don't always work out as you expect! You will still be getting to know the garden, the lay of the land, the microclimate, and the needs of the people using the garden. It's best to be as flexible as possible. Always be prepared to change and adapt your plans. This is especially true of a training garden where new features are constantly being built just to show people how to do things – one bright spark once suggested we put wheels on the trees because we moved them round so often – and to keep providing interesting work for people, so as to engage them.

Tilling the soil to remove weeds and stones can be a back-breaking task, and it is a commitment to the future, as is building compost heaps to feed the soil. There is a wonderful metaphor in compost making; it takes the waste products of the garden and transforms them into the life-giving material that feeds the soil, all the creatures within the soil, the plants we grow, and ultimately ourselves.

Putting in stakes and supports is a commitment to the future too, and some plants will need support throughout their entire lives, but what a crop they will yield if you do that properly!

After you have lived in the garden through the four seasons and have discovered the plants that grow there, you may feel ready to make long-term plans for their care. This might involve some study, as there could well be plants that you know little about. You might find yourself talking to other gardeners, reading up, and visiting other gardens so as to discover the best way to look after them. You will be clearing away any rubbish, dead material and noxious weeds to make the growing area clean and hygienic. You will be testing the soil, and thinking about what you are going to grow, and why, and where to put it.

PRINCIPLES OF PRACTICE

In any therapeutic or community garden, it is usual for people to come to an agreement on the qualities and the commitments that they want to prioritise. In the gardens I have worked in, these have been considered important:

- To garden organically – no chemicals, good compost heaps, focusing on a healthy living environment for plants (and people)

- To develop a beautiful and productive teaching garden that people would be proud to work in

- To be open to the public

- To work to the highest horticultural standards, regardless of the diverse background of the volunteers

Volunteers should be allowed the opportunity to do all the jobs in the garden, with supervision if required, regardless of ability. Of course, safety must be taken into consideration. Some limits have to be imposed if, for example, people suffer from blackouts or epilepsy, or have very poor balance; they should be discouraged from working at height. If some people take a bit longer, need more supervision, or don't do the job as well, then so be it. People should not only be allowed to make mistakes but should be encouraged to do so. Process is more important than product.

A commitment to involve people as far as possible does not, however, mean always involving people in all decision making. Managing a large therapeutic garden and estate with twenty to forty volunteers (some of whom might be very unwell and most having no background in horticulture) as well as a staff team, is a complex task requiring specific skills and knowledge. It is important to be clear which issues can be brought to the entire team for discussion, and which have to be managed by the manager or staff team, who have the relevant experience.

While there is a commitment to encourage everyone in the garden to have a say in the running of it, volunteers will be encouraged to take on responsibilities only as and when they feel ready for it. Many people come to a garden with considerable skill sets and are much more able to carry out some projects than any of the staff team. Great examples of this were a joiner who completely refitted a kitchen, a plumber who fitted new toilets, artists who led groups to complete wonderful projects, and IT gurus and journalists who between them transformed publicity materials. Then there were social workers and teachers who developed induction programmes for new volunteers in the garden.

As the work of designing the garden progresses and deepens, we can gradually develop the Principles of Practice, not just for the garden itself – organic, open to the public, etc. – but more importantly for the people working there. These are just as relevant to community gardens as therapeutic gardens.

People can stay in the garden as long as they feel they need to, i.e. volunteer placements should not be time-limited

In the same way that physical illness might only last a month or take several years to recover from, leaving a legacy of vulnerability, the length of time needed to recover from mental health problems also varies. Time available should not be limited arbitrarily. The possibility of returning must be allowed, should the need or desire arise. People often said that just knowing they could come back to the garden if they needed to enabled them to continue working outside of it. (The exception is in children's gardens, where age appropriate progression is expected.)

Be open minded and optimistic about what people can achieve, no matter what hurdles they face

Let everyone have a go at everything (so long as it is personally safe for them to do so) and remain hopeful of personal recovery.

Allow people to participate in activities that appear potentially risky

The best example of this is using machinery for strimming and hedge cutting. All staff and volunteers have to be well supervised and given the appropriate training, and there have to be no medical issues to prevent them from doing it safely, as discussed above.

> During one meeting, in which we were trying to decide on the most important principles of the garden, one woman said she wanted to have a quad bike to whizz around the garden on. I was taken aback by this one, as we were

working in a garden of just over an acre, so long distances were not involved. People laughed and thought she was joking, and I tried to wave it aside, but she was adamant. It took a while to unpick what she was getting at but eventually it was this very issue. She did not want to be limited to nice, safe jobs all the time because she had a mental health problem. She wanted to be allowed to take calculated risks in the same way that everyone else did in life.

At one point, a number of people got involved with forestry work, and this included funding for six people to attend a chainsaw course. Understandably, there had to be some serious thinking around the safety aspects of this and whether the garden should be responsible for letting people go ahead with the course, but the point was that the volunteers would be subject to exactly the same standards during the course as anyone else. If they passed the certificate, they would be just as qualified. Our only concession was that all participants – staff and volunteers alike – would be supervised by someone on site who had many years of chainsaw experience. The people who completed that course gained so much in confidence in all areas. By confronting their fears in one aspect of their life and managing to overcome them, these people gained the confidence to tackle other challenges, such as attending group courses, flying on a plane, dealing with stigma, etc. In actual fact, and according to statistics, the most dangerous tool in the garden is not a chainsaw or another power tool, but the ostensibly innocent ladder.

Making time for talking and listening should always be a priority

The process is more important than the end product. The garden creates its own deadlines in terms of seasons and growth, and if the project is part of a much bigger organisation, external agendas can also be imposed upon it. This can make it easy to lose sight of the priorities, which should always be about the people. With someone who may have never had a voice or ever felt they have been truly heard, it's important to listen carefully when they do start to talk. You will only get one chance to get it right. They are unlikely to try again if they feel you didn't listen the first time.

To see change as a positive thing that allows growth into our lives

This might have been the hardest concept for us all to grasp.

> After one particularly busy season in the garden, a valued and able member of staff pleaded with me not to take on anything new. "Could we please just stand still for a while?" I had to answer no; with new arrivals and the constant need to adapt, as well as the pressures of making sales and securing funding, we had to always be advertising, raising our profile, and moving forward. I did, however, recognise that he had worked very hard and was tired. We came up with the solution that staff would take turns to run a small John Muir[8] Award group (a lovely conservation course) out in the back field, every Friday for six weeks. They all loved doing this and it gave them a bit of a respite from the daily run.

Most of us, especially if we have been unwell, tend to fear change greatly, for it has usually been negative changes in our lives which have brought us so low. It was therefore important to foster the understanding that if everything stays the same then we will all stay the same too, and there will be no opportunity for anyone to feel better. We have to recognise that learning to do anything differently can be hard work and uncomfortable.

Value everyone's life stories

When we meet people for the first time in any walk of life, quite often their behaviour doesn't make sense to us. Maybe it's the young woman who jumps every time anyone walks behind her, or the person who carries his belongings in a big heavy rucksack on his back all day and won't put them down. When we find out that the woman was routinely abused by a member of her family and goes through life perpetually terrified, and that the young man grew up in an institution where his personal belongings were constantly stolen or ransacked, then we understand and have every sympathy.

Strive to establish a culture of openness, honesty, clarity and mutual respect

Hold site meetings regularly. I was very fortunate to have had three years of professional group-work training as a community education student, which helped me facilitate groups like this. This can be hard for new people to get used to and it often takes a long time for them to participate, but almost everyone joins in with the right encouragement eventually. It may not be the most popular event of the week or month for some, but I always feel it to be the most important. People may have spent a long time in hospital wards, or in an oppressive school, workplace or family, where they got very little say in how things were run and what treatment they received. They may not be used to being listened to or asked for their opinion. Great care has to be taken to make a meeting safe. Ground rules have to be firmly agreed on, established and adhered to. These include respectful listening, constructive criticism only, approaching topics with sensitivity, and accepting that people all learn and absorb information at different rates and in different ways. You can explore many different techniques. A talking stick can be passed round when things get a bit heated. You can use paper cut-out red herrings which are raised when people wander off topic, and you can have a ranting box which people can stand on for five minutes to air something that is bothering them. Some of the volunteers themselves will have had prior experience of managing groups, and we can all learn a lot from each other.

> During one particular meeting, the discussion became heated and it was getting harder to control the group. One man taught me a lesson I'll never forget. He put his hand up to speak, and instead of asking people to stop raising their voices and talking over each other, he surprised me by saying: "This seems to be a really important issue; clearly people have a lot they want to say. Can I suggest we have a ten-minute break, get some fresh air, perhaps someone could make a pot of tea and we can come back to it once we've all had some time to reflect?" This was pure genius, and I copied him many times.

Celebrate achievements

This applies not just to the high-flyers but to everyone. It might be a simple achievement like arriving on time for a week, doing a good job of cleaning duty, or staying for the whole hour during a site meeting. With children, it could be something as minimal as getting through five minutes without interrupting. John Muir training is excellent because it does not give certificates for high levels of competence, but simply for involvement and commitment to completing the course. It is accessible to everyone regardless of ability, and it might be the first certificate some volunteers have ever achieved.

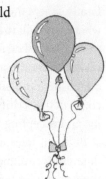

Establish a culture of shared responsibility

Giving people responsibility is not only great for their self-esteem but also a necessity in making the whole project function. When decisions are within your making, try to involve people as much as possible. For example, what new garden feature people might like to build? How would people like to be addressed: service user, volunteer or member? How many open days should we have? Children could make a joint decision on where they should go on their bike ride or work out how to take fair turns of a special piece of equipment.

Many agencies claim to do this but it's easier said than done. I found that it took a lot of time and work. For instance, if you are planning to discuss a complex topic at a meeting, such as feedback on welfare reform, then people usually benefit from getting to know the subject over time. Introducing a topic at a meeting cold doesn't work well for most people. It helps to approach it in different ways. Background information can be given out in written form ahead of a meeting. Bringing up the topic as you work alongside people in the garden ahead of the discussion helps to introduce the subject in a casual setting and gives people time to mull it over and ask questions. Having two or three meetings instead of just one helps most of all, as people can digest the information in the way that suits them best, have time to think it over, and come back with their reflections.

Measuring progress

Most therapeutic gardens depend on external funding and understandably, agencies and funders often want to see some evidence that their money is being used effectively. However, progress in mental health is often complicated to measure and it is certainly not a case of 'one-size-fits-all'. The most genuine measure needs to be personal, qualitative and subjective, and even then it can be hard to define. I would find it difficult to define progress in my own life as there are so many external influences.

If someone begins their time in the garden feeling withdrawn, isolated and unable to give voice to their problems, then turning to a GP or a psychologist, or taking medication might be considered progress for them. For someone else, this might be seen as a backward step. Agencies often try to capture progress for the funders by using surveys. A good survey would allow the participants some input into the questions being asked. They would need time to prepare for answering the questionnaire, opportunities to do group answers after discussion, and possibly people to support them through the process. A simple, multiple choice tick-box type of questionnaire is easy to produce and collate but it often catches very little of the true picture.

I did conduct one major survey of the garden, in which I tried to ask open questions about how people felt about various situations.

For example:

- Has your level of confidence changed? Can you give an example? Is there anything else you would like to say about this?

- Has anything changed in how you manage at home? Can you give an example? Is there anything else you would like to say about this?

It took months to prepare people for. We discussed and amended the questions in advance, then we provided one-to-one support for individuals completing it and offered group facilitation for joint responses.

It was not a process you could repeat very often because of the time involved, although I did get a lot of help from very skilled volunteers. However, it was an immensely satisfactory exercise as we gained useful insights into what worked for people and what we needed to change.

The best place to be even on the darkest days.
Response from a volunteer

KEY POINTS

Preparing the growing environment

- Good support leads to productivity.

- Listen, read, ask questions, visit other places, and keep learning.

- Process is more important than product – encourage people to make mistakes.

- Change, however challenging, brings the possibility of better things.

- Involve people meaningfully in decision making where possible. Where necessary, teaching people the skills to take part and have their say.

- Measuring progress is subjective and nonlinear; it is not a case of one-size-fits-all.

CHAPTER 3

SEED SOWING

Sowing seeds is the most magical process in gardening. It is very special to hold a seed in your hand and know that its whole DNA and the blueprint for its life is contained within it, no matter how tiny it might be. You sow, you tend, you wait, and if you are lucky, magic happens! My favourite seed is the sea bean. It travels on ocean currents, often for thousands of miles until it finds a suitable place to germinate, to release the life so tightly packed within its tough shell. It is heart-shaped, the colour and texture of a conker (horse chestnut) and fits exactly into your hand. I like to give them to people to have in their pocket so that when they feel panicked or alone, they can wrap their hand around it and feel connected to the whole process of life.

Seeds come in a huge range of sizes, shapes and textures, and they all need different conditions. Some are so small that you need to mix them with fine sand when you scatter them on the soil; the sand lets you know where you have sown them, otherwise they are difficult to see. Others, like peas and beans, are bigger, so you can push them straight into the soil. Some like to be covered, some like to sit on the surface, and some germinate within days while others might take months or even years. There are those, such as lavender, verbena and evening primrose, that need to experience winter conditions (either by sowing them in late autumn or by putting them in the fridge for a time) before they can germinate. This is nature's way of making sure they have made it through the cold weather before they put up tender shoots. Many crops go to seed quickly (that is, they flower and then when the flower dies, they set seed for the next season) and move on to the next stage in their life cycle. When salads have flowered, for example, they are no longer so good to eat. So it's important to re-sow these crops at regular intervals to ensure an on-going crop.

Once they germinate, certain seeds hate being disturbed, which means it's better to sow them into biodegradable containers like cardboard tubes, either singularly or in little groups of two or three. Then you can plant the whole thing, tube and all, when the seedlings are strong enough to survive outside. Peas and beans often do better if they're sown this way. Other seeds like marigolds are very gregarious and don't mind being scattered straight onto the soil in large groups.

You have to be careful you don't sow seeds too thickly, or when they germinate they are too crowded and are prone to diseases such as "damping off" (a fungal disease). Thinner, regular sowings produce better results.

Getting seeds to germinate involves constant problem-solving. You have to ask yourself lots of questions before you sow. What kind of soil does the seed require and how deep should they be planted? How much water, heat, and light does it need? Is it the right season, and so on and so forth? This process takes you out of yourself and opens your mind to lots of possibilities, before you've even considered the creatures that might eat your seeds and the measures you should take to prevent them.

It is a wondrous thing to put seeds into the ground and watch them grow. Yet people often approach it with scepticism and a lack of confidence in their abilities. It can seem like a strange, fiddly job, and people new to the process often do it without much faith until they see the results. When they spot them, those first shoots fill people with such satisfaction. Many people are so delighted by the vegetable crop they have produced that they will eat it every day for the whole season – boiled, baked, mashed, fried, raw!

Sowing seeds also buys you some time. Working with someone who is constantly troubled by suicidal thoughts can be a frightening experience for everybody. I have very seldom met anyone who truly wants to die. However, I have met many who find coping with life extremely hard to bear. I used to dread Friday afternoons (we closed at weekends) because there was often someone who would come to talk about feeling so suicidal that they couldn't get through the weekend. I had to establish that I respected their feelings, but that I did not agree, nor could I help them with that plan of action. I would, however, be happy to help them make a plan to get through the weekend instead. I would offer to talk to them about it again on Monday or refer them to agencies who might be able to help over the weekend.

You can look at the resources available to someone feeling suicidal. Often, the person will remember what has been helpful in the past and will be able to offer ideas. Not going into the weekend with nothing to fill their time can be the main one. The weekend can feel like a big yawning chasm. People can feel completely paralysed and unable to make the simplest decisions. So, think about a plan, even a simple one. What will they make for their tea when they get home? Do they have a TV programme they like, a crossword puzzle to do, a friend to call? Can they go to the library on Saturday and look up whatever they are interested in or complete a research task that will help the garden? Can they go for a nice walk somewhere on Sunday or are there any free exhibitions they can visit? It is often the big empty space that is so hard to deal with. Making plans collaboratively is also a better way to ask for help. People, sometimes even professional support staff, get scared or can even seem angry when someone talks to them about feeling suicidal, as it can feel like a frightening responsibility. However, most people will respond more positively when asked if they can help someone plan how to survive.

If I was able to get someone with suicidal thoughts to plant something like potatoes or beans, sometimes I managed to plant an idea as well (obviously after getting to know the situation and establishing some trust). We would make a kind of deal that works like this:

> "I can't imagine how much pain you must be in for suicide to seem like a good alternative to staying alive. However, if you work with us until these potatoes/beans are harvested and postpone the decision, then in October you will still have the same options, but you might feel differently."

It sounds too simple, and obviously I have condensed the conversation somewhat, but it has always seemed to work. People really do want a break from these thought patterns, and putting a visible time frame on it seems to makes it possible to do so, at least for a bit. By acknowledging that it's their decision and that you respect their feelings, you are leaving that option open but are asking for just one season to see if things improve. It gives everyone a chance to relax a little bit. Constantly working with suicidal thoughts is exhausting and frightening for the individuals concerned, and for those working with them. With that little bit of breathing space, the garden and the people in it can do their work and, with luck, come the harvest, more than just potatoes will be growing.

SOWING THE SEEDS OF AN IDEA

Once someone has begun to feel safer in the garden and is beginning to trust the people they are working with, you – friend, support worker, colleague – can begin to sow some seeds of hope that might take root and grow into helpful ways of thinking and behaving.

You might try exploring an issue such as lateness:

"I've noticed that you seem to find it difficult to get to work/the garden on time in the morning, and that this is upsetting for you."

"Do you know what is causing you to be late?"

"Are you finding it hard to get to bed on time and to get to sleep?"

"Are you waking up on time but just finding it too difficult to get out the door?"

"Are you finding it takes you a long time to decide what to wear and that this is making you late?"

"Are you finding the bus journey daunting?"

"Would it be helpful to look at some sleep hygiene ideas? Some people find it helps if they drink less caffeine, stop looking at screens mid-evening, and get more exercise during the day."

"Would you like me to give you a call in the morning to help you get out of the house?"

Some people say they just get paralysed with anxiety and can't get out the door. Often, it helps if I suggest what they are going to be doing when they arrive, so that they can focus their attention on that rather than the journey.

> "Would it help you to text me if you're feeling panicky on the bus, and I could call you and talk to you during the journey?"

Or if tiredness is the issue:

> "I've noticed that you often say you feel tired and that you find it difficult to do the more physical jobs. This isn't unusual when someone is feeling anxious or depressed because those emotions are exhausting, but there might be some ways to help. Why do you think you have no energy?"

> "Shall we look at some ideas that might help you feel more energised?

> "Could diet changes help? I could help you focus on that or put you in touch with a dietician?"

> "Do you think it might help to work on some exercise routines? Perhaps get some support to attend a gym or join a walking group?"

Or if it's to do with smoking:

> "I've noticed that you have a lot of smoking breaks. If you would like to try and get that under control, or even to stop smoking, I would be happy to try and help."

"It can be very hard to give up on your own, but people are often successful if they get support."

It is worth noting that there seems to be an interaction between nicotine and some antipsychotic drugs[9]. Smokers often seem to need higher doses of these drugs in order for them to be effective, which can result in more side effects. Conversely, stopping smoking can sometimes result in a reduction of medication.

Or managing emotions:

"You have said you find it difficult to manage your anger/depression/fear. If we put our heads together, we could perhaps make a plan for when you're feeling overwhelmed?"

"Can I give you something to read? Do you think you would like to attend a support group that might teach you some strategies for coping with your feelings? There are several groups that happen locally, which people say have really helped them. Would you like to buddy up with someone?"

"Would you like to work on some protocols with us so that we can catch these emotions early before they escalate? If you feel yourself getting angry or overwhelmed, you might ask for a different task or for a rest or a short walk to make you feel calmer?"

The immediate answer might well be no, but the seed has been sown. There is help available and when the person is ready, they will often come back and say, "Well, actually, I've been thinking about what you said last week/month/year, and I would like to try that now."

I worked with Jenny for many years. She had been drinking steadily since she was a child, copying her parents. She knew no other way to cope with life. She was a great gardener and a loyal, trustworthy friend and colleague, but when the working day was done she would buy her alcohol on the way home and the rest of the day and night was a blur. Her future looked bleak because of her poor health and declining ability to function day-to-day. Her loneliness was devastating. She felt too ashamed to open up to people about her drinking. She did not want to be a burden and tried to cope on her own.

I tried everything I could think of over the many years she worked in the garden; information on agencies that helped with alcohol addiction, offers to accompany her as she visited them, affirming our confidence that, with help, she could tackle this awful disease – but to no avail. I think it was only our strict rules banning alcohol on site that sustained her by giving her a break from its hold for a few hours each day. As she went down this hellish spiral, we began to lose hope for her survival.

Then, one Monday she came into the garden, looking a bit more sprightly than usual. She said: "I've stopped drinking. I went to see my doctor on Friday, and he gave me some tablets [to prevent withdrawal seizures] and I've stopped drinking." We were absolutely gobsmacked. She was resolute and did not touch a drop for at least six months. She then had a few short relapses but they only lasted for a few days and she managed to get straight back on track. Her health did improve, although the years of drinking had taken its toll. Her strength of will and commitment astounded us all.

SEED SOWING

It was like the sea bean, the time and place had to be right. After being buffeted by the waves for decades, the seed of hope finally put down roots and started to grow. She taught me a valuable lesson in not giving up on people; it had to be done in her own time and in her own way, and this process takes as long as it takes.

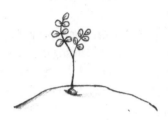

KEY POINTS
Seed sowing

- Gardening involves lots of problem solving, which leads to a more open, flexible mind.

- Investing energy in seed sowing and planting encourages people to think about the future and its many possibilities.

- When everyone works together on a problem, everyone invests in the solution.

- Some ideas can take a long time to germinate. Don't give up: hold on to hope.

CHAPTER 4

PLANTING OUT, COMPANION PLANTING

When it comes to moving plants out of the greenhouse and into the ground there are a number of factors to consider. Are the plants hardy enough to survive outside? Is the weather right? Do you need to harden them off first – to gently acclimatise them to outdoor conditions? Where is the best place for these plants to grow? As with sowing seeds, you need to consider wind, sun, shade, shelter, and aspect (north or south facing?). Spacing is also important, as you need to leave enough room for them to grow but not so much that it allows weeds to shoot up in between.

All plants are different in the amount of space they need between them. Cabbages, for example, are normally planted 18 inches to 2 feet apart, whereas peas quite like to be in triple rows, 3 inches apart, or round a wigwam-shaped structure of canes or willow. It is not widely known among non-gardeners, but some plants grow much better with specific companion plants growing close to them. They protect each other and shelter each other, and, in some cases – we still don't really know why – their presence alone helps the other to thrive. Some plants will do well in their allotted spot in the garden but will need to be brought back into the shelter of the greenhouse as the weather becomes colder. If looked after in this way, they will be able to go back outside again the following spring, vigorous and healthy.

Sometimes, young plants have been compromised by their nursery conditions. It's common for people to be given beautiful flowering plants for special occasions, such as Mother's Day or Easter. The plants look great when they are bought and for the first week while they are still flowering, but they often fail to thrive when they are planted into the garden. The nursery may have forced them to grow unnaturally, by withholding water and nutrients so that they flower early for those special gift days, which can cause the plant to become distressed. It could then be sold in a supermarket without being hardened off properly (acclimatised slowly to living outside), so that when you plant it out it becomes unwell and needs a lot of attention to nurse it back to health.

It's clear that the plants grown in the best conditions when young, which are only moved out into the garden when they are ready, are the healthiest.

PEOPLE MAKE FRIENDS BY DOING THINGS TOGETHER

If you work with a group of people in a garden, you will get to know each other very quickly.

I once asked for volunteers to move a big boulder from a nearby field into the garden and place it into the rock garden we were building. I thought this was difficult and not a job I would have considered to be much fun. I immediately got six volunteers who rushed off to inspect the boulder and started to figure out how to manoeuvre it. It took them all afternoon. They ended up filthy and exhausted but with a huge feeling of satisfaction, and they got to know each other in a way that sitting in a meeting room for months would probably have never achieved. They had to talk to each other. It was dangerous, as the boulder was heavy. They had to pay attention to each other, look at each other, listen to and watch out for each other. They got to know who was good at keeping the morale up when they were flagging, who was good at the technical stuff like using rollers, who was strong, who told jokes and made them all laugh, who gave lots of encouragement, and who went off and brought back tea and biscuits when they were getting tired. Best of all, they had a bond and a great memory to talk about for weeks afterwards.

Remember these are mostly folk who are really struggling to connect with others and are fearful and anxious around people. They might typically walk with their heads down, trying not to catch anyone's eye or engage in conversation. What an achievement to manage all of that co-operation. How wonderful to suddenly realise that you have made it through an entire afternoon without worrying about all your personal stuff.

Like plants, people have different preferences regarding how much distance they are comfortable with when standing beside another person. You will recognise that feeling when someone stands too close to you and you begin to feel claustrophobic and have the urge to move back. Similarly, if someone stands too far away, that can feel awkward too. A comfortable distance between our self and another is often dictated by life experience, by cultural background, and by our relationship to them. Understandably, if you have had your trust betrayed, it might be harder for you to stand close to someone, especially a stranger.

Somatic Experiencing™[10] is a body-based approach to shock and stress disorders and is the life's work of American psychotherapist Peter Levine. This approach aims to safely release traumatic shock that has become frozen in the body at times when it has been over-whelmed. I found it useful for learning how to listen to my body better and how it reacts to discomfort, and how to protect myself from situations that make me feel stressed. A simple exercise you can try for yourself to find the edge of that slightly uncomfortable feeling is around social distance. Ask someone to stand about six feet away and slowly walk towards you. You will notice a slight sense of alarm in your body – I feel it in my stomach, a kind of tenseness – when they start to get too close for comfort. It may not be too close for them, however.

It's useful to repeat the same exercise with you approaching them, to see if the space differs. If you can hang on to the memory of that feeling of unease, it's a useful guide when you are working with trauma. I will often be listening to someone's distressing story and suddenly become aware of that feeling and, as often as not, I will discover that I am leaning forward, bent over, head low, mirroring the body language of the person I am talking with. It is a timely reminder that I am allowing their experience to affect me in a way that is too personal. It is their story not mine, and in order to support them effectively I have to maintain a safe distance. In this instance, I will remind myself to sit back in my chair, breathe deeply and slowly, and try to make sure I feel fully calm myself so that I will be in a position to help them out of their distress.

By becoming too close, I can disable myself. It's a bit like finding someone in quicksand. If you wade in to try and help them, then it's likely you will start to sink too. It's better to find a way to tie yourself to an anchor and throw them a lifeline as you talk them out of their panic, and to encourage them to be still. You metaphorically stretch out your hand to pull them out. Compassionate and caring people who don't learn to protect themselves in this way when working with trauma (as a friend or in a professional context) can often be affected by what is usually known as 'burn out'.

It is always interesting when a new volunteer comes into the garden who likes to hug people. Many of us hug our friends when we meet them, but you've got to be aware that for some people this will feel intrusive and threatening. Lots of places have all sorts of rules about not having any personal contact, but they sometimes just don't work. For some people, there seems to be a real need for that contact. It's good to have a discussion about it. Gradually, you can develop a code of conduct based on respect, watching for cues and gaining consent.

SPEND TIME WITH THE PEOPLE WHO MAKE YOU FEEL BETTER

"A friend is someone who thinks you are a good egg even if you are slightly cracked."

Companion planting is a fascinating subject. I met quite a few people who came to the garden from various psychiatric hospitals who seemed markedly reserved when it came to mingling with others. They had been advised in the hospital not to mix too much with the other patients, nor to get too attached to them, and some had a real resistance to being classed as a 'patient'. At the same time, there were others who made lifelong friends in hospital. Companion planting is a useful metaphor. I want to grow beside people who like me, trust me, have confidence in me, and believe in my ability to flourish – people who value me. It doesn't matter what their role is, be it friend,

family, patient, volunteer, colleague, doctor, manager, director. For me, a good companion plant is someone who makes
me feel good about myself and helps me to think positively.
Most people come to share this belief. In the garden it is always
humbling to see how hard people work to be good companions
to one another, however distressed they may be in their personal lives. Though coincidental, I often think about how the
extraordinarily diverse mix of people in a garden helps with
this process.

I came into the garden one day in early spring. The ground
was warming up and everything was starting to grow, but
nothing was ready to eat. Many of our volunteers had personal 'allotments'. These were small patches of ground in
which they could grow whatever they liked, as distinct from
the communal beds of the garden. Nearly all the volunteers
had strawberry plants. Imagine their delight when they
checked their allotments one day and each of them found
a big, ripe juicy strawberry on one of their plants (at least
a month before the fruiting season). One of the volunteers,
who was a bit of a joker, had snuck in early with a punnet of
store-bought strawberries and put one on each plot. Little
details like this would make the day go better.

At one point in my career, I had a very severe back injury
which kept me off work for about six months. When I
returned to work, I was very weak and could only carry
a half-sized tray of seedlings. It was around that time that
Dona started in the garden. She was very shy and very
strong, and she liked to do simple repetitive jobs. She had
come to the garden because she had become depressed at
not being able to find any work. She did need a little more

instruction and support than most. I asked her a few times if she would mind being my back for the day to help me work in the garden. She loved that role and I think she benefited from the extra attention she received and the sense of purpose it gave her. I relied on her to help me with tasks I could no longer manage. We became a great team for the long months it took for me to recover. I gained enormously from her strength and patience and enthusiasm – and she had the most wonderful smile. She felt valued and gradually her depression left her (as did mine) and her lovely sunny nature shone through. We were perfect companion plants.

Therapeutically, there are lots of benefits to working with people in a garden. Rather than working one-to-one in a standard therapy session, you can see how people interact with others and give them useful feedback. Ideally, if someone has both kinds of support, then you can work even better – giving feedback that allows someone to go to an individual therapy session with something concrete to work on. Then the person can come back to the garden having worked out what she or he wants to practise.

Sometimes it's hard to recognise that people are expressing their companionship.

Martin (and many like him) always wore a baseball cap in the garden. He would come in through the gates with the cap pulled low over his face, looking down at the ground, turning his shoulder away from anyone he passed. He tried to draw as little attention to himself as possible. It felt like he wanted to be invisible and avoid contact at all costs (for good reason, as he had been subjected to unwanted attention and abuse in the past).

After a few months, he asked to speak to me and said he needed to leave the garden, as nobody wanted him here and they would be better off without him. I could see he genuinely believed this, but I did not. I asked him why he felt this way and he said he "just knew" that was what they were thinking. I accepted that that was how he felt but disagreed that there was any evidence for it. I told him that nobody had made any complaints about him or requested not to work with him. When asked if he had any evidence other than his feelings, he said everybody avoided him; nobody ever came up and spoke to him. I said I could understand that, and he might well be right about their behaviour, but I thought he was wrong in thinking he knew their reasons.

Grabbing a baseball hat, I walked past, emulating his body language, and asked him how he thought I looked and felt. Martin said I looked sad. I asked him if he would approach me if I looked like that, and he said he wouldn't because it seemed like I wanted to be left alone. Light bulb moment! I explained that I thought he was wrong about how people felt. When I saw him walk into the garden, I often felt I would be intruding if I approached him. I suspected others felt the same. Far from ignoring him, they were being very respectful and responding to his signals, which meant they cared about him and did not want to upset him. We agreed that he would give it some more time and that he would try to change the messages he was giving out.

I asked Martin to stop half way down the drive on his way to the garden in the morning, think about how he was presenting himself, look up at the first person he met and say,

"Hi, how are you today?", and then come and tell me the response. It was a risky, frightening thing for him to do but he recognised that if he wanted his life to change then he had to learn to do things differently. I had great faith in the other volunteers to respond to him with friendship and support as they all knew from personal experience just how hard it was, and how much of an effort he was making. It was not a quick fix and he stayed in the garden for several years. He was fortunate to have some one-to-one support from time to time, where he could practice little strategies of his own. Gradually things improved for him, and in turn he offered a lot of support to other volunteers coming into the garden.

KEY POINTS

Planting out, companion planting

- You get to know people quickly by working alongside them; not just their difficulties but also their strengths.

- Study and learn your own emotional reactions so that you get better at controlling them and not letting them take over.

- Seek out people who make you feel better about yourself – just like companion plants, which help one another to flourish.

- Gentle honest feedback, coming from a place of objectivity and kindness, can help people understand their own behaviour and other people's reactions to them.

CHAPTER 5

WEEDING AND MULCHING

If you want to grow crops in the garden that are healthy and vigorous then you have to keep them free from the weeds that will steal their light, nutrients, and growing space. A weed is just a plant in a place you don't want it to be. Some you will want, like nettles, as they are nutritious and beneficial to insects, but they still need to be kept under control.

Some people love weeding and get great satisfaction from kneeling all day close to the earth, pulling out the weeds and leaving nice, clear rows of plants with lots of room to grow.

There are little shallow-rooted annual weeds, like chickweed, which are very easily pulled out of the ground, and these can be added to the compost heap to be turned into valuable feed for the following year. Unfortunately, there are also very tenacious weeds such as ground elder, creeping buttercup and bindweed; these have widely spreading roots that are difficult to remove and can completely infiltrate the garden if unchecked.

Once weeds have taken root, you need to keep on top of them year after year. No matter how much work you put into digging them up, you have to be vigilant, checking regularly for any signs of re-emergence. There are also deeply rooted weeds like docks, which can grow large and be difficult to remove. In attempting to dig these up – to literally root them out – you can cause disruption to the soil and damage to nearby plants, as their roots are often entwined. You have to be careful you don't dislodge the plant you want to protect. After you've pulled them up, don't put pernicious weeds on your compost heap but in an appropriate place where they cannot seed or take root.

Some people hate weeding with a vengeance and would much rather be doing exciting, energetic work like creating a new bed, cutting down trees or turning over big heaps of compost. In an organic garden, it is usually accepted that it is almost impossible to be completely weed free. The ones to concentrate on are those that threaten the growth of what we want to cultivate. We can be tolerant of the odd shepherd's purse growing on the edge of the cabbage patch or daisies in the lawn. It's not just about appearances, it's about how well everything is growing together as a collective.

I have noticed an interesting phenomenon over the years when weeding beds of cabbages. Once you've planted the bed, cabbages usually grow quite vigorously by themselves. The gardener can then move her attention elsewhere for a bit. When she returns to the cabbage bed a few weeks later, she discovers that the cabbages are strong and robust and growing well, but that the bed is full of weeds which, if left, could end up competing with the cabbages for space. Following the conventional wisdom, she then weeds the bed and thinks all will be well. The next day, she comes in to have a look and discovers that the pigeons have had a splendid dinner and shredded the cabbage plants. The weeds may have been competing with the cabbages for space but for a while they were also hiding them from the cabbage-loving pigeons. Weeding can be a bit more complicated than it looks.

After the ground has been prepared, the plants put in, the weeds taken out, and everything is watered and fed, it is time to apply a mulch. This is usually a thick layer of well-rotted compost or leaf mould. The mulch helps to keep in moisture and stops the plants drying out. It also helps to stop the weeds growing back, and it slowly releases nutrients into the soil to feed the plants. Regular application of a compost mulch keeps soil and plants in good health.

EMOTIONAL WEEDING

The things which inhibit and hinder our mental and physical health and our emotional growth – the weeds, if you like – can sometimes be the same things that protected us during traumatic events. It can be difficult for us to see that if we are to thrive as our lives and needs change, so must our habits and ways of thinking.

The 'weeds', that is, the beliefs and habits that might be holding someone back, may have long vigorous roots stretching right back to a childhood when they were abused, bullied or neglected. The beliefs developed at that time through these damaging experiences can be invasive and have a strong hold on people for the rest of their lives. Many people carry feelings of guilt, perhaps remembering: "It's all your fault. You made this happen"; or of toxicity, thinking they can affect others through their presence alone: "You will make your mother ill if she finds out". If told to them by adults, children often assume these lies are true. People often try to stay out of harm's way by keeping a low profile, by staying as invisible as possible. Never getting dirty, always completing house work, never answering back or questioning anything; these things might work for a child trying to avoid the attention of an abusive adult but they do not work so well for an adult trying to make their way in the world. The loneliness and isolation caused by hanging on to such secrets is very hard to live with.

In order to survive, people might develop habits of self-harming, substance abuse, overworking, under- or overeating, as ways to escape the pain they are feeling or to comfort themselves in dark times. They might have come to believe it was better to keep important information such as a history of PTSD (post-traumatic stress disorder), depression, anxiety, panic attacks or even dyslexia, secret, by never making a mistake, and trying to become invisible. In the past, when they had tried to share their story, it had always led to disbelief, bullying, threats or distress. As with weeding, great care must be taken when approaching deep-rooted habits.

Substance abuse may be a way of self-medicating for seemingly unbearable traumatic memories. Self-harming, which from the outside appears destructive and counterproductive, might actually become a way for someone to stay present. Instead of going into a trancelike state where they fear they have no control over their actions and end up harming themselves even more, the individual self-harms in order to feel something other than complete numbness. It might be their way of returning to full consciousness and the present. It might bring them back from that frozen state where they were unaware of their body and what it was feeling. If it is the pain of cutting that helps someone stay present and makes them feel safer, then the individual could be encouraged to work on other ways of achieving this outcome that are less harmful, like substituting ice for a blade. The experience will still be painful and achieve the same goal, but it will be less damaging. Self-harm is a very complex subject with many different causes and outcomes. What is clear is that if it does seem to have a purpose then 'weeding it out' needs to be done very carefully.

In the short term, even if some self-harming habits appear to serve a purpose, there is no doubt that it would be a better long-term goal to learn to manage without them. Often these habits have outlived the traumatic situations they were established in, but they still leave permanent scars. If someone has survived trauma and the danger has passed, their task would be to learn to live with the memory of it, without resorting to survival techniques that, although useful at the time, do them damage.

People might also, through low regard for themselves, have developed very poor habits of self-care. A common scenario when people are very distressed is for them to go home at the end of the day and just sit immobile on the sofa, getting stuck there for hours. They don't think to turn on the light, put the heating on (if they can afford it), switch on the kettle for a hot drink, prepare a wee snack, and listen to the radio or play some music for company. The habit of neglecting their own well-being can become so deeply ingrained that these small steps will never occur to them; not until they can weed out the thoughts that are saying: "I don't deserve to be looked after, comfortable or well-nourished". Changing our habits, especially habitual ways of thinking, takes hard work and perseverance. People have to have something bigger than themselves to work towards in order to make that huge effort seem worthwhile. Being a team member in a beautiful, productive, inspiring garden seems to be able to provide that bigger purpose. They become part of a creative process and work towards building something positive.

"I can't get out of bed for therapy but I can't wait to get up and put my work boots on."

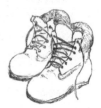

When someone has been deeply traumatised by early life events, especially abuse, it can sometimes take many years, even a lifetime, for them to find a place and time that feels safe enough to talk about it. Very often, part of the abuse involves terrorising the child into keeping it secret with the threat of terrible repercussions if they speak up. As a child you have no way of judging how likely that is and you believe that adults are telling you the truth, no matter how bad. Having carried these beliefs and fears right through our childhood, they become entrenched in our thinking and are hard to combat as an adult, even once the threat seems to have disappeared.

I suspect when you have lived in fear of someone for many years you can never truly feel completely safe. One strategy people use in order to keep what happened to them a secret is to develop a protective shell, pretending to the world that it never happened, which seems to become harder to manage as they get older.

Beth described it as wearing a tightly buttoned up overcoat to hide what was going on underneath. As the years went by, it seemed to get tighter and tighter until it became far too hot and uncomfortable. She longed to take it off but was too scared. After working in the garden for some time and starting to feel safer there than she'd felt in a while, she realised the coat had got so tight that the buttons were beginning to pop. She didn't open them deliberately, they just burst open, and she began to tell her story. You would expect her to feel relieved to be free of the constraints of her protective shell, the need to constantly pretend everything is ok. Instead, she said she felt very naked and exposed, as though all the world could see her distress, which was indeed very evident.

> At this point, the garden and the people in it had to wrap round her like mulch to help her feel safe and protected. As she grew stronger, we were able to help her knit a new garment to live in – a comfy frock, one that would enable her to recover, to move about freely and easily, and to live the life more like the one she'd always wanted.

In a caring community, people have a lovely way of comforting someone when they are distressed. It is quiet and unassuming. It takes the form of stopping by with a cup of tea when they see you sitting alone, offering warm smiles of greeting when you arrive, leaving you a seat by the door at meetings so that you can escape easily if you need to, bringing a little bit of extra lunch to share with you if you don't think to bring any, and watering your plants when you're having a bad day and can't come in. Small, simple acts of care can mean so much to someone when they are low, especially if they have known few expressions of kindness. Because the other people in the garden might have had similar experiences, or at least know what a bad day feels like, they can be wonderfully adept at being attentive without being intrusive. Some gardens do actually knit patchwork blankets to wrap around people when they are feeling particularly vulnerable. People love them; love the weight of them, their warmth, their bright colours, and the fact that they have been made collectively by their friends in the garden.

I often came into contact with someone who had very low self-esteem. I don't mean the lack of self-confidence that many of us experience in certain situations, but a deeply rooted belief in their own worthlessness and inability to get anything right. It is very upsetting to hear someone express such beliefs when they seem to be a kind, caring, skilled, and eminently valued and valuable member of the team. After working successfully, sometimes for hours, they might make a wee mistake and hurl abuse at themselves:

"I am so stupid."

"I always make a mess of things."

"I can never get anything right."

It is clear they have come to believe such negativity about themselves. I used to think that lots of encouragement and constant affirmation would improve matters:

"You did a good job there."

"You do have lots of skills."

"Of course people want you to be here."

The trouble was that it just didn't seem to work. The feedback I got from some people was that it actually made them feel worse, as though I was not listening to them or believing them, so they refrained from talking about their feelings at all.

So, instead, I found it better to focus on giving people as many positive experiences as possible within the garden. Encourage them to look at the successful results of their labours:

"Do you like the way that bed looks now you have finished planting it?"

"Do you think that that apple tree will do better now that you have pruned out the dead wood?"

Encourage people to live in the present rather than viewing themselves through the prism of the past. You can help them to look at the evidence of their work and express it in their own words:

"Yes, I actually quite like the way that bed looks."

"Yes, it looks a bit healthier already."

People are more inclined to believe what they hear themselves say than what you tell them. The day-to-day living together also helps, due to the gradual process of feeling accepted perhaps for the first time through the approval and companionship of peers, and of sharing a purpose that is greater than any individual.

Being part of such a focused community acts on the individual a bit like the mulch does in the garden, which unobtrusively protects the plants from the ravages of harsh weather, keeps the weeds in check, encourages the roots to grow and slowly improves the structure of the soil and its nurturing abilities.

KEY POINTS
Weeding and mulching

- If we don't pull out at least some of the weeds, there isn't room to plant what we want to grow.

- Some weeds are very deep rooted and dislodging them should be tackled with great caution.

- Self-harming habits might serve a purpose initially, so forbidding them outright can leave an individual vulnerable to greater harm. Less harmful substitutes can be useful until the person is strong enough to manage without them.

- Self-inflicted wounds are every bit as painful and distressing as accidental ones.

- People need a lot of comforting, reassurance, protection, kindness and support when they are going through the process of disclosing trauma.

- Just being there and listening are very effective ways of supporting someone.

CHAPTER 6

THE GROWING PROCESS: WAITING AND WATCHING

You have to be patient. Some plants grow quickly and produce an abundance of fruit or flowers, which you can harvest within one season. Others need to be left to grow in their own time.

I love asparagus. When you plant asparagus, you are creating a bed that will be productive for years to come, one which will require a lot of work, watching and waiting. You have to dig the ground well and incorporate lots of manure and compost because asparagus are heavy feeders. You usually have to send away for the plants, as they are not so readily available. You have to water them faithfully, feed them well, mulch them as they grow, keep them weed-free and then, after all this work, you will see the first shoots peeping through the ground.

Your mouth begins to water as you see how fresh and delicious they look. Do you pick them? No, you don't. Asparagus gets a bit traumatised by being moved so you have to leave them that first year to develop root systems and build up their strength. This will lead to an even stronger crop in the years to come. If you harvest them that first year it will weaken them and they will not yield as well as they might in the future. They require a lot of work but if you like the bounty of fresh asparagus, they are well worth the effort.

Being patient is part of the growing process. You can't rush it; recovery and growth have to happen in their own time. You might even decide you want to grow a tree from seed, maybe a hazel tree so that your children can harvest the nuts, which will take ten years or more.

Gardeners know that during the growing season, you have to constantly observe the plants. How much have they grown each day? Do they need more or less water? Are they showing any signs of deficiency? Are they infested with aphids or mites? Are the birds, rabbits, or slugs trying to eat them? Small adjustments must take place day-to-day to keep them thriving.

Lots of things happen on a daily basis when a large group of people are working together in the same space, as is the case in therapeutic and community gardens. A garden is dynamic. The plan for the day can change at the drop of a hat, and if you want people to have a voice in what they are doing then you have to be prepared for a bit of anarchy. Things happen all the time that you can't plan for or predict, and there is always the balance between the needs of the people in the garden and the needs of the garden itself. This can create a bit of pressure for everyone, which is both challenging and useful at the same time. This is exactly the right dynamic and it is what makes working in a group so stimulating and organic.

People often talk about the unescapable pressures and timelines that have to be met in the "real world" outside the garden, for example in the sphere of business. So, it is actually useful that the garden imposes some pressure too (even if a garden is much more forgiving). For example, in the height of a wettish, warm spell in summer, the grass will grow quickly and if you miss a cut or two it can become too long for the mower to manage, which in turn will lead to lots of extra work with strimmers, mowers and raking off the cut grass.

THE GROWING PROCESS: WAITING AND WATCHING

If you lose a bed of seedlings because no one gets round to weeding or watering them then it could be too late to re-sow and that crop can be lost for the season. The growing process has its own rhythms which cannot be ignored; the garden is alive and has its own deadlines which have to be met. The whole team has to be prepared to run with that, but you can't always expect people to fall in with your plan without a reasonable explanation of what needs to be done in the garden and why, and why now.

In the same way, there is a rhythm to recovery. Grieving, for example, is a process. People understand this when they lose a loved one but often don't realise that they also have to grieve the loss of a limb, an ability, perhaps through illness, the loss of a career, or perhaps the loss of family life after a divorce. It makes it very hard to calibrate recovery and growth as these do not move in straight lines. Instead, they have peaks and troughs. In some ways it is similar to physiotherapy, when the work can seem like agony at the beginning and does not feel like progress at all.

The recovery process is also about the often hard-won growth of understanding. At one point in the garden, the volunteers were slow in getting back to work after the morning break. Gina, the person leading the group planting brassicas (the plants of the cabbage family, such as Brussels sprouts, kale, cauliflower, etc.), was getting impatient as they were in the middle of a job that had to be finished that day, which included protecting the vegetable patch with netting to keep out the hungry pigeons. These pigeons were poised and ready in the trees, waiting for us to go home. She had told people break was over and folk were still dithering, so she went into the shed and starting shooing people out,

71

and as she passed the toilet door she knocked and said break was over. Eventually, everyone went back to work, not noticing the incident.

Sometime later, Graham, the person who had been in the toilet, came to find me and was very upset indeed. He had been frightened by the banging on the door and was now very angry that someone in this therapeutic garden could be so insensitive as to do such a thing. He never wanted to work with Gina again. I tried to reason that Gina had not meant to subject him to anything upsetting but was just trying to get people out into the garden, probably because she was getting a bit anxious about needing to finish the netting before the end of the day.

In site meetings, we had discussed at length about how breaks were long enough for people to use the facilities. He then told me harrowing stories about his child-hood with abusive parents and siblings who did not allow him any privacy even in the bathroom. They would constantly barge in, terrorise and humiliate him. He 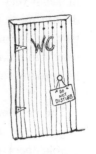 hated using bathrooms outside of his own flat and only did so when absolutely necessary, and preferably when no one else was around. I said that now I knew the circumstances, I understood better how upsetting the knocking on the door must have been. I asked if we could speak to Gina together so that she would understand too. It took some time to persuade him, but he agreed. I then went and gave Gina a brief outline.

At first, she was quite put out, as she didn't think she had done anything wrong. I was able to persuade her and once she was sure she was calm enough and in control of her own feelings, she came and listened to what Graham had to say. When she heard his story, Gina too was horrified at how she had unwittingly upset him, and she was humble enough to admit to that. She offered her profuse apologies and promised never to do it again. She said that if Graham found it easier to use the bathroom during the working sessions, then she would see to it that no one interrupted him.

Far from Graham's original claim that he never wanted to work with Gina again, their relationship improved greatly in terms of trust and mutual understanding. Both Graham and Gina were brave enough to face up to criticism in a positive and constructive way, over what seemed at first glance like a fairly trivial issue, but which was in fact quite complex.

OUR OWN PERSONAL GROWTH

For most of us who go into therapeutic work of this kind, we start off with the idea that we are there to help other people with their problems. We don't expect to have our own behaviours placed under scrutiny. It can be a steep learning curve when our actions as group leaders are not automatically supported and we are expected to examine them, realise we could have done something differently, and learn from that to improve our practice. We expect the people we work with to be able to do this, but somehow we sometimes don't apply the same expectation to ourselves. It can come as something of a shock, as few people enjoy criticism, no matter how constructive the intention. The notion of 'same rules for everyone' should be a strong maxim in the garden in many different settings.

I believe this to be one of the main values of a garden that makes it feel safe for people, especially those who have grown up with adult carers they could not trust. As adults working together it is OK to disagree, OK to criticise behaviours, OK to challenge rules and instructions, so long as you are willing to talk it through with the people involved. It is not OK to make comments about people which you are not prepared to defend, explain, or discuss with the relevant party. In other words, gossip is certainly not acceptable. We all learn continually through this growing process, even if it isn't always comfortable.

Allotments are a good example of this. As previously mentioned, we decided to offer all of our volunteers a small allotment – a little patch of land – in the garden so that they could grow whatever they wanted to in their free time, albeit still within the open hours of the garden (lunchtimes, before we started work for the morning, and a half hour at the end of the day). The idea was to help people feel 'rooted' in their own space for a period of time. It began to work too well; soon I noticed people were beginning to plant fruit bushes, flowering shrubs and bushes, which were only suitable for long-term ownership. I felt that some people grew so attached to their allotments that they stayed in the garden even when they were ready to leave, all because they didn't want to give up their piece of land. I suggested that we limit what was grown in allotments to herbaceous perennials and annuals (vegetables and flowers), and that people cleared their allotments by the end of the year and were assigned a new allotment in the New Year.

While people did recognise how attached they were becoming to their allotments, there were a lot of complaints about this suggestion. We had a site meeting where everyone got to have their say. Then we decided to have a vote. Needless to say, I lost, and the old regime of keeping the same allotment continued against my better judgement. However, having opened the discussion, I then had to abide by it. I had to remember the principle of not asking for people's opinion if you are not prepared to be changed by it. It was a steep learning curve for all of us. I had to stand by my promise to go along with the decision of the group, even though I believed it to be a problematic one, and to move forward with the consequences of that decision.

SOMETIMES THE CONDITIONS FOR GROWTH HAPPEN ALMOST BY ACCIDENT

One day in the garden, I was working with a wee group of volunteers in a greenhouse potting up seedlings. Jenny had been there for a few months and was settling in well, and Morna had just started that day and was clearly very nervous. We were working together, chatting quietly, telling stories and getting on with things, when there was a bit of an emergency elsewhere and I was called away to attend. I asked Jenny if she would look after the new recruit, Morna, and left them to it for a short while, confident that she would do a good job. When I came back, they were managing beautifully and seemed quite relaxed. I asked if they were OK and as they all seemed quite happy, I left them to it, popping in now and then to check on them.

At the end of the day, Jenny asked to talk to me. She said that when I asked her to take over she had been nervous, but then she'd thought about how much support people had given her when she first started and how scared she had been. She realised that Morna was probably feeling like that now, so she rose to the challenge and did her best for her. Afterwards, she said she felt proud that she had been trusted to look out for someone else and felt really good about herself for being able to offer support.

MEASURING GROWTH

When you spend a long time working on the same piece of land, you learn where the sun shines, where the shade is, which bits get wetter and which bits are warmer. As expressed in the preceding chapters, the beauty of spending a lot of time with people in a work-focused setting is that you get a much better idea of how capable they actually are and what their skills are. With this in mind it is useful to suggest to any volunteers who are supported by psychiatric services (which are inclined to focus more on symptoms), that they are welcome to invite them into the garden for medical and psychiatric reviews, instead of conducting these in the hospital where they usually meet. It gives the 'patient' a chance to host the visitor. This means that they can choose the space – either one of the meeting rooms, or even out in the garden – offering teas and coffees if they want to. They can show the psychiatrist or psychiatric nurse round the garden, pointing out what they have been working on, talking about future plans for the garden, and introducing them to people as they wander round. Similarly, it can have the same effect when someone invites a family member or friend to visit the garden. They get to see a different, sometimes more confident and engaged side of that person's personality than they might be used to at home.

It can make a huge difference to their relationship with the psychiatric staff, who are often astounded by the difference in the way the individual is presenting, and how skilled and capable they seem to be. When you go back to the hospital, it's hard not to turn back into a patient. I have accompanied people to hospital reviews and watched them change into somebody I didn't recognise on the way up the drive. Their body language switched from open and confident to power-less and subdued in a matter of minutes. I don't mean to say this was the fault of the hospital staff, it was more about the institution; it is designed to help people who are unwell, and so on entering it people subconsciously adopt that persona.

It is an alarming lesson on how expectations can affect people. I sometimes think that what works for people in a garden is the fact that it feels like there is just so much work to do. People see quickly that they have to muck in and start to take some responsibility if we are going to keep the show on the road. At other times, of course, I am not so positive about that situation.

GROWTH CAN HAPPEN SLOWLY

The other benefit of spending many hours a week with people over an extended period of time is that you notice the small, incremental changes in their behaviour that are not obvious to them. When someone despairs that they are never going to get well, you may be able to point out that you can actu-ally see some improvement. It is not always obvious what an improvement looks like to people. (See the section on *The Tidal Model* in Part Two, page 210.)

A common step forward for many people, for example, is the ability to cry.

THE GARDEN CURE

I had spent a lot of time with Freddie and had listened to him tell the sad and distressing story of an abusive childhood. He told his story over several weeks without a trace of emotion and seemed very distanced from it, while at the same time terribly affected by it. I came across him one day, sitting in the middle of the lawn sobbing his heart out. I bent down to comfort him but he said he wanted to be left alone, that he hadn't been able to cry since he was quite a young child, and that it felt like something he needed to do alone. It was a fairly common story. Sobbing for hours on your own doesn't seem like a step forward, but for many people it was just that. The growing process can take many different forms.

KEY POINTS

The growing process: waiting and watching

- Sometimes, all you can do is be there and be present for someone, and that can be enough.

- Progress doesn't always make you 'feel better' at the beginning. Progress doesn't take a straight course but occurs in dips and surges. Recurrence of symptoms is not a failure but just a stop on the way. Don't lose heart.

- Complaints don't need to be bad. If managed with patience and clarity, they allow each party to gain a better understanding of the other.

- You need to work on your own well-being continuously in order to support others.

- The same rules and behavioural expectations should apply to everyone.

- Expect more! High expectations encourage people to try their best and achieve more.

CHAPTER 7

COMPOSTING

Making compost is a kind of alchemy. You take all the weeds, kitchen trimmings, vegetable waste, grass clippings and spent matter from the garden, give it a good stir, cover it and leave it to cook for a season. All the work goes on under the cover, the worms and other creatures play their part and, lo and behold, it turns into gardener's gold – a fragrant, crumbly, dark brown material that feeds the garden, the soil, the plants and the creatures that live in the earth together. It is the transformation of garden and kitchen waste into a hugely valuable and much sought-after product.

In the first walled garden I worked in, the soil had been fed and nourished for a hundred years and was rich and dark and loamy. You could run your hands through it and just feel the fertility. You could dig down for two spits (a spit is the length of a spade) and it was still the same; a gardener's heaven, easy to dig, full of nutrients and worms, yielding and abundant. Imagine my dismay when I went to work in another beautiful old walled garden to find I was working in sub-soil – the layer usually well below the productive surface – full of boulders with no life in it at all. The topsoil had been removed for sale and the garden was stripped bare. It was backbreaking work to dig it over, and for the first few years the main job was to remove rocks and steadily build up compost with whatever we could find.

This would become the heart and 'powerhouse' of the garden. Gradually, slowly, as we tilled and fed it, it began to regain heart. It was a very misleading garden. It looked as if it was a couple of hundred years old, going by the age of the walls, but in fact, as a growing space, it was very new. A garden is only as old as its topsoil, as many buyers of new houses find out as they try to grow in builders' rubble.

Compost is the engine of an organic garden. It is often assumed that it feeds the plants like chemical feeds claim to, but in fact its purpose is more to feed the creatures in the soil and improve the conditions for them to live and work and multiply in. Sure, you can add NPK (nitrogen, phosphorus and potassium) fertiliser to the garden to feed the plants, but it will not feed the worms (which produce wonderful, nutrient-rich worm casts) and other creatures that are essential to keeping the soil alive. It is a bit like the way we bring up our children. We can either feed them low-value processed food and top that up with vitamin pills, or we can give them a wholesome, wholefood, balanced diet. You can take them to a gym to exercise, which works in some circumstances, but they won't get the sunshine and fresh air they'd get from running around in the park, walking along a river, or working in the garden with you. Perhaps, most importantly, they won't get that connection to nature, or to you. Compost also conditions the soil. It introduces air and bulk to a heavy clay soil, helping it to break up and drain better. Compost adds water-retaining texture to dry sandy soil. It adds all the necessary nutrients in exactly the right proportions. You can't just keep taking things out of the soil. You have to put that energy back in, and nature will help you do that if you let it.

There are many parts to the process. You need to collect all your materials: weeds, kitchen waste, plants that have died back and finished their annual life cycle, cuttings, grass clippings, etc. The different components have to be mixed together

– wet grass can be mixed in with leaves and dry stalks so that it all rots down better. Bulkier material can be shredded to make it compost faster. The heap is built and then most gardeners would try to turn it over at least once during the year to mix air through it again. The finished product is then 'riddled' or sieved to take out any bits of plastic, metal or glass that may have snuck in, to make a mulch feed for the beds or potting compost. It's strenuous work but a glorious process. Many people especially love the tasks involved in tending to the compost – the gathering, building, turning and riddling. They are often delighted by the black, sweetly fragrant end product.

COMPOSTING TURNS USELESS WASTE PRODUCTS INTO A VALUED AND VALUABLE COMMODITY

I love compost. It's the perfect metaphor for the recovery process. When people arrive in the garden for the first time, I greet them and we have a wee chat before I take them for a wander round. If they have come to the garden because of depression or anxiety, I try to ask them what they want from the experience, rather than how they are feeling – which can sometimes take people to the sad place they are trying to get away from. Often, people will say they want to get back to where they used to be. In time, they will understand this to be both impossible and not actually a good idea, as that was what led them to where they are now.

On our tour, we pass the compost heaps. It is general good practice to build three compost heaps. The first one is where you put all the fresh garden waste, the second one you leave for a season to cook, the third is usually about two seasons old, and its contents are ready to use.

When I show people the first heap and explain its purpose, they sometimes say things like: "That should be me in there, I am rubbish, and people think I am a waste of time". Such is the persistent stigma of having a mental health problem, often coupled with unemployment, that people do genuinely feel like they are society's rubbish and are unwanted and unvalued. It is truly distressing to hear someone talk like that. One woman actually very perceptively described herself as feeling "not valuable" – a slightly different nuance to "not valued". When I looked up the words in a dictionary, "valued" was defined as "highly regarded or esteemed", while "valuable" means "worthy of respect, admiration or esteem, of use, service or importance", a subtle but telling distinction.

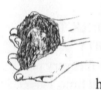

When we move on to the third compost bay and take off the cover, new people are usually amazed to find the rich, sweet, fertile material, transformed from the rubbish. We can then have a conversation about how we hope they won't go back to feeling the way they did before, but would progress to be more skilled, content, and feel valuable and valued by society. People find it hard to hear that kind of talk when they are feeling anxious or depressed, but the story of the compost sticks; the image of rubbish being transformed into gorgeous valuable compost is embedded into their thinking.

Fortunately, we live in a society that appears to love gardening. There are endless TV programmes on the subject, and it is now deemed a valued occupation. On stepping into the garden, people can change their role from mental health 'service user', unemployed and unwell, to gardener, and that alone is transformational. Imagine the difference to casual conversations in the pub, when you meet someone who asks what you do and you have two options:

"I've been having mental health problems…"

Or:

"I work in this fantastic garden…"

If you choose the second response, your sense of social status takes a leap up the ladder and you begin to receive some positive feedback and to feel better about yourself.

I imagine few people would introduce themselves as a mental health service user in the pub, but at least they no longer have to lie or hide the reality of what they are living through. They have a choice of what they say depending on how they feel. Working in horticulture is a positive activity, which people are interested in. They'll soon be asking you about the best soil for their roses. It doesn't matter if you don't know the answer, as you are still learning.

Twenty years ago, if I went to a social event and someone asked me what I did for a living, the conversation would usually peter out quite quickly if I said I was the manager of a mental health service. If, however, I said I managed a beautiful garden that has lots of volunteers and is open to the public, you could guarantee there would be a lot of interest. Thankfully, mental health has entered into the media and public discourse much more in recent years. This is thanks in part to well-known figures being willing to discuss their own experiences, such as Monty Don and Princes Harry and William, who all shine a spotlight on mental health issues. However, although great progress has been made in recent years and there is a more commonly held understanding that mental ill-health can affect anyone of any standing, individuals can still feel ashamed and stigmatised.

When people are new to gardening, they tend to overlook compost heaps as a pile of rubbish. However, once they work in the garden and they understand the process of turning garden waste into a truly remarkable, life-sustaining product that is in high demand (we were always being badgered by the public to sell it), some people really become invested in it.

One of the side effects of psychiatric medication is often alarmingly quick weight gain. It is not unusual for people to put on two or three stone (up to twenty kilos) in six months, most noticeably round the middle. This in itself can be severely depressing and disabling for people. Doing exercise for its own sake doesn't work for lots of us, but once people get the compost bug, they are willing to undertake the work to reap the reward. Turning compost heaps is great for building upper body strength, while riddling is good for reducing the waistline. When it is done as a team it is much more enjoyable and less daunting. There is a sense of purpose and the stronger people support the weaker until they build up their strength.

Ian came to the garden having had a stroke which left him with a weakness down one side. It affected his balance and made bending and working in the garden difficult at first. The inactivity of a long recovery had made him put on weight. He discovered composting and began to notice that all the riddling he was doing was beginning to reduce his waistline. It meant a great deal to him to become stronger and fitter, and to find something he could do, even if it was slow-going at first, which produced such great results.

COMPOSTING

Jenny, with a similar history, became completely captivated by the composting process. She became a real expert and went on to work in several other gardens, advising and helping them make great compost. Her enthusiasm for the subject was so infectious that when people were shown round a garden full of beautiful plants and abundant fruit and vegetables, she would capture them with such passionate explanations of the importance of compost that it was often the compost they left talking about at the end of the day.

Margaret, who had a history of trauma, loved using the garden shredder to prepare woody and sometimes thorny material for the compost heap. There was something about being allowed to work the powerful machine – the rhythm of feeding it and the quality of the result – that seemed to soothe, energise, and inspire her all at once.

The nature of the task also helped her to work closely with at least one other person, which she usually found difficult. She had to wear a face guard, ear defenders and protective gear (which rendered her blissfully anonymous, like wearing an invisibility cloak) but she still needed to be aware of others working or passing nearby.

The focus required for feeding in prickly branches, for having to work in rhythm with the person passing her bundles of brambles and woody materials, and above all, for piling the sweet smelling results in another layer on top of the compost heap, was to her, as she often remarked, some of the best therapy she'd experienced.

I like to believe too that as people are exerting a lot of physical energy in making compost, they are, at some much deeper level, recognising the transformational process of turning waste products into a richly valued one. Without realising it, they start to understand that anyone coming to the garden feeling like 'rubbish', like a waste product of our society, can also be transformed into someone who feels valued by and valuable to society. After expending all that energy to feed the soil, they might also get the message that it's worth thinking about how they are feeding themselves.

KEY POINTS
Composting

- Composting transforms materials often discarded as garden waste into rich and valuable material that makes the garden grow.

- Composting takes a long time; producing anything of value demands hard work.

- It shows people who feel useless and discarded by society how they can achieve a sense of purpose.

- The ensuing sense of value of the end product attaches to the person producing it.

CHAPTER 8

MAINTENANCE, TOOLS, AND TRAINING

While some jobs in a garden are exciting, like sowing seeds, planting out, and harvesting fruit, much of the work is house-keeping. You need to keep the garden clean and clear of rubbish, mow the grass regularly, trim the hedges, sweep the paths, and wash the pots and greenhouses. If you fail to do these things, the garden gets cluttered and can become dangerous, causing trip hazards and accidents. Piles of weeds or plant material left lying about will encourage slugs and snails. Holes in nets and fences will allow the birds and rabbits to eat your crop. Dirty pots will encourage disease in your plants. It's just like housework. You need to establish a routine for maintenance and cleaning to keep the garden healthy.

And then there is the matter of using the right tools for the right job. If you want to do fine pruning, for example, you need sharp secateurs which are in good working order and not an old pair of blunt shears. There are some tools specifically designed for certain tasks, such as a sharp half-moon for edging grass. Some of the very best tools, if used with care and looked after, are infinitely adaptable. The kirpi, which is my favourite, is a light and versatile Indian hand tool that can hoe, weed, dig, and cut. Of course, all the best gardeners are also addictive scroungers and improvisers. They can often be seen rummaging through skips and various building suppliers' yards for pallets, wood, containers and the like, to put to good use in the garden. In my early days, when there was very little money for the garden I was working in, I had to resort to old pairs of net curtains to keep the cabbage white butterflies off the brassicas. They worked beautifully and looked rather charming. Having good tools and keeping them sharp and clean is an essential part of gardening maintenance but so too is keeping a lookout for anything else that might come in handy to help the process. You must be ready to improvise if an opportunity presents itself.

People also need regular and repeated training on the correct use of tools, as even the simplest, most commonly used tools can be dangerous. Ladders, used regularly in gardens and in the home, cause more accidents than any other tools. It's easy to become complacent when you become overfamiliar with something.

HOUSEKEEPING SKILLS

If you have a lot of people working in a garden, then you have to establish a way of managing the shared living areas. The toilets and eating areas need to be cleaned regularly to avoid disease. The floors need to be swept and washed, bins need emptying, dishes need washing, and so on. In order to achieve this in a big project that does not have the budget for cleaning staff, all the participants – including any paid gardeners and instructors – have to take turns at doing this work.

Sometimes people coming to therapeutic gardens have had very difficult childhoods where the living space was not maintained well, and they never had the chance to learn this kind of routine housekeeping. Other people have completely lost confidence in their ability to complete even simple tasks successfully.

So, asking people to do a half-hour job in the living areas can be much more fraught than you might think. On top of that, you might have people who, as a symptom of their distress, have become very worried about dirt, infection and disease, and will want to have every surface thoroughly disinfected. If they work alongside someone who really doesn't know or care about that level of cleanliness, it can be challenging.

First of all, people have to understand and accept that the work needs to be done, and that there is no one else to do it but ourselves. Put simply, they then need to turn up and complete the tasks or the system falls apart. It takes more management than you might think. Some people might need a great deal of support to learn how to do some of the tasks. For others, such as those who have experienced overly critical or punitive parenting, schooling or workplace environments, they need support to simply face the prospect of doing a job so publicly. They might believe they will be criticised for doing it badly, which can make them feel exposed. It helps if more confident and sympathetic volunteers buddy up with people who are feeling vulnerable. In a garden which is also a mental health service, people quite rightly expect to be supported on a bad day. But, unless their distress is very severe, for that half hour of domestic chores, they have to put their distress on hold and get on with it. It might sound harsh, but learning to put your own stuff aside for a short time in order to contribute to the group is a necessary and rewarding step forward. At the very least, they will go home feeling like they have accomplished something that day, even if it is just washing the dishes.

MEETINGS

Earlier, I discussed how difficult it is for some people to attend a meeting with a large group of people. Again, that fear of being criticised or made to look stupid can be quite overwhelming. Some people have to start from outside the open door, before gradually moving to the doorway, to a seat right by the door, to a seat beside a trusted colleague, and so on. Some will last only a few minutes before they have to take a break, gradually extending the time they can manage. With support, patience and encouragement, I have found that everyone usually manages to attend meetings in time. More importantly, they will be able to have a voice in those meetings as well. The only thing that is non-negotiable is that people have to start somewhere in the process, even if it's just standing outside near the door; they can't just opt out altogether. This again might sound like a hard line, but it is an important part of believing in people. Believing that the individual will eventually succeed in attending will help them to do it.

The ability to attend a meeting is a powerful social skill. I have been at hospital reviews for a single patient with over eight people in attendance. A large group meeting like this can prove nerve wracking especially when the subject under discussion is the person's own behaviour and future. Some people have children and are expected to attend parents' meetings or have problems with addiction and want to attend AA or similar group sessions. Meetings come up all the time. If you want to participate in a political democracy or even just have a say in your own welfare, you have to be able to attend collective discussions.

Of all the learning in the garden, the ability to lead a more orderly life and be able to speak up for oneself, are often the most difficult. But it can make the real difference to people, especially when they have grown up with chaos and have never had their feelings listened to. Taking charge of the little things, being able to negotiate who does what and keeping the place clean, helps people get closer to managing the more complex issues, like family or group relationships.

One of the simplest tools for supporting people that I have found, is the giving of feedback. When you spend a lot of time with people several days a week, you notice slight changes in their behaviour that they might not be aware of themselves. They may not realise that, although they are still in a lot of pain, they are actually making progress. People might begin by working mostly by themselves or on the edge of a group while their body language paints a picture of loneliness, isolation and fearfulness. Three months later, they might be tearful and want to talk for long periods of time, and this is progress. At this point, they will not feel better. However, from the outside it is apparent that there has been some movement; they are not stuck, and the journey of healing has begun. It can really help someone to hear this first-hand.

When I was in my late thirties with my severe back injury, I couldn't do anything for weeks except take strong painkillers, which knocked me out, and lie in bed feeling miserable. One day, I was crying and raging to my husband about how awful I felt and how bad the pain was, and he replied that actually he thought I was getting better. My response was total incredulity. "How can you say that?" He replied that I hadn't even been able to moan about it a month before. He was right, and it helped to hear it. No matter how small my steps were, I was moving in the right direction.

TRAINING

In a therapeutic garden, where many people are experiencing deep distress, how do individuals keep themselves safe, sharp and fit for purpose? Regular training is helpful, and this can take many forms. There are, of course, the standard basic training days that many agencies offer. These can be a good start but they usually fairly basic as they are often aimed at beginner level. A great deal of the best, most appropriate training I experienced was introduced by the volunteers themselves. If someone finds something helpful and makes a reading suggestion, buy a book on it for the library and, if possible, attend or run a short course for people in the garden. In this way, everyone can learn and practice together. These can be vital tools which help us maintain, sharpen and further our skills. They are discussed in greater depth in Part Two, 'The Tool Shed'.

It's good to keep a library on site covering, as well as gardening, all aspects of mental health and well-being, which will be well used, and people are often very happy to donate a book they have found helpful. Sometimes being introduced to a new understanding, insight, technique or way of thinking can be truly life changing.

During days working together in the garden and in site meetings, people will often bring up issues which are troubling them; not sleeping, loneliness, poor diet, negative self-talk, suicidal thoughts, and worries about medication. If a few people are interested, this can become a short series of weekly discussion groups on a particular topic. Once again, talking to one another is essential in helping everyone understand the issues at play, and also for sharing solutions. One in four people seek help for mental health problems in this country. I firmly believe that everyone should have access to training and literature on mental health issues – not just mental health professionals but also people experiencing them, and anyone interested. We all spend a lot of time with each other in gardens, groups or in social situations without a mental health professional present, so, as already discussed, it's important that we all learn how to approach mental health problems, in the same way that medical first aid is rolled out to the whole population.

The other tool for better practice is reflection. Most days, I will arrive at work and hit the ground running. I might have to sort out a work programme, prepare budgets, complete orders, deal with visitors, and talk to new volunteers who are about to start. I love it all usually. But every so often a day will come around when I will arrive at work and, for some reason, I just won't know what to do. None of it seems to make sense. I wander round the garden, observing what is going on, drifting apparently aimlessly and somewhat uncomfortably. I used to call them my 'chocolate teapot' days.

I am usually back on form the next day, and for a long time I didn't understand what those days were about. Eventually I began to realise that these moments were really valuable. These were days when I would step out of my daily routine and look at what was happening with a new perspective; I would take some time to wonder what it was all about, and why we were doing what we were doing. This was the time to spot the strengths, the gaps in my knowledge, and the possibilities; the time to accept that I needed to think about the direction I was going in. Sometimes, these days give me the opportunity just to chat and listen to people. I recommend them to anyone who feels caught in a treadmill and has forgotten the direction they are meant to be heading in. Take a day off and play in the garden. It will pay dividends in productivity.

THE GARDEN CURE

It sounds very mundane, and perhaps a bit boring, but in a life made chaotic by a lack of structure in the early years, or following the disabling effects of mental illness, or just the ever changing nature of life, the very routine of the garden itself can be really helpful. The hygiene, tidiness, regular feeding and watering, the routine checking that everything was functioning well, the regular repairs – which in gardening terms we call 'husbandry' – is a major ingredient in helping people get their lives or their thinking back in order. This is not rocket science, nor is it a quick fix. But, bit by bit, learning to look after the garden, the plants and the living space spills over into people's own lives and improves the quality of their time at home.

KEY POINTS

Maintenance, tools and training

- Tools work best when they're in good condition; to achieve this they need constant maintenance and sharpening.

- You are the most important tool in use when you are working with other people. Your behaviour, attitudes and values can have a big influence on others.

- Contributing to the collective welfare of the group helps people feel useful and needed.

- Start with what you can manage; it doesn't matter how distant it might seem from your end goal, so long as you make a start.

- Information about mental health should be accessible to all, not just to the medical experts. Everyone gains insight from learning through experience.

- It is good to have a day off; step out of your routine, observe what is happening around you, and ask questions. Take a breath of fresh air and get a new perspective.

CHAPTER 9

SUPPORT AND PROTECTION

Some plants are half-hardy. This means that when it is warm and mild these plants will thrive; they will produce beautiful flowers and plentiful crops. But, when the temperature drops in winter, they must be taken inside and protected in order for them to survive.

Some plants grow happily on their own, without much support at all. Others, while they can grow unaided, will produce better fruit if they are given the right support. Left to their own devices, tomatoes will grow along the ground and produce hundreds of tiny fruits. But if you provide a stake to support them, if you protect them from frosts, remove the side shoots, and limit the amount of fruiting trusses they produce, and feed them well, you will be rewarded with big juicy, delicious fruit.

Sweet peas can be left to grow along the ground too, but you will get fewer flowers, a shorter flowering season, and they will be spoiled by the rain and mud. If, however, you make a wigwam of several canes for them to grow up, pinch them out when they are small and take off the seedpods as they develop, you will grow beautiful fragrant flowers exactly at eye height which will bloom the whole summer long.

Cabbages, on the other hand, don't usually need staking. They tend to look strong and robust but this is misleading. They need to be protected by a little collar at the base of their stalks to keep cabbage root fly at bay (which try to burrow down and eat the roots) and also a net to keep the cabbage white butterflies from laying their eggs on them, and pigeons from feeding on their delicious leaves.

Some plants only need protection or support for a short period of time, a few months or a season, while others will need it for life. It pays to provide for this by putting up polytunnels and greenhouses to protect from cold weather, and fruit cages for berries with structures and netting over the brassicas, and stakes for trees that will last the lifetime of the plants. If you do this, they will yield plentiful crops for many years to come.

WHO NEEDS SUPPORT AND WHAT SHOULD IT LOOK LIKE?

The garden leader also needs support. She needs proper breaks, as gardening can be hard work. She needs to be able to make plans and have the equipment and funds to carry them out. She also needs security of tenure. You can't plan a garden for one season. Instead, you plant trees for your children and grand-children. Once you have planned and planted the garden, you can't keep changing your mind and moving things around, or the plants will not thrive.

In my experience of working in therapeutic gardens, where all the volunteers arrive with a background of mental health problems, I've learnt that while everyone has a different story there is a shared understanding of what a bad day can feel like (but this is likely to be the case in any social group). This includes the staff team. In other words, we are all invested in creating a safe place in which to work, learn and live together.

As with plants, people don't all respond to the same kind of support, and every individual needs a different package. When

SUPPORT AND PROTECTION

I first started working with trauma, I found music worked very well with one person in particular; it helped to form a link between us. The right music was able to calm her, distract her and take her to a safer place. The next person with similar issues, to my dismay, didn't respond to music at all and found it annoying in the background. However, they were able to work really well with imagery and symbolism.

> When James was distressed, it was obvious to everyone on site. He would sit alone in the middle of the garden and would be so visibly upset when anyone approached him, that several of the volunteers came to where I was working to express their concern. This happened many times. Usually, if someone was able to spend some time talking to him, he would be able to settle his feelings and calm himself enough to go to work with the others. When I asked if he really wanted everyone to know how upset he was, he said emphatically that he did not, but that he wanted key people to know. After I explained how visible his distress was to the other volunteers (I was not saying that there was anything wrong with it, but just wanted to check that he was aware of the effect it had on other people), he agreed to work on ways to communicate how he felt without it being so obvious to everyone on site. He began to avoid 'broadcasting to the nation' as we came to call this, when he really wanted to send a private call. We hatched a plan whereby he would wear a certain colour if he was having a bad day and needed to speak to one of us. We agreed we would simply acknowledge the colour he was wearing, 'nice jumper', and at some point in the day one of us would come and talk to him. This enabled him to get to work when he came in, confident that when the others were set up for the day, and

when someone had some time, they would come and find him. Quite often, by the time we got around to asking him if he would like a one-to-one chat, he would say he was all right and didn't need one. The garden had worked its magic.

In the same way, people will often begin to feel safe and part of a community in the garden, but when they get home, they will lose that confidence. Old feelings of panic and isolation creep back in. It sometimes helps to give people an object from the garden, perhaps a pretty stone, a pinecone or a big seed (like a sea bean) to put in their pocket as a symbol of connection. When they are home alone, they can reach for the object that connects them to feeling safe.

Support can come from many different sources, just like the sweet peas with a whole circle of canes. These canes – or the people and activities that support us – are essential to us all. But often when people become mentally unwell, they lose contact with friends, colleagues and family. They may need some professional support for a while. You might have at least ten canes in your circle: a GP, a psychiatrist, a support worker, medication, a garden (if you are lucky), the close friend who is always there for you, the sister who meets you once a week to go swimming, the acquaintance with whom you go for walks or to the cinema, the man who says hello every day when you are out walking your dog, the woman in the newsagent who always has time for a chat, the Samaritans at the other end of the phone when you feel overwhelmed in the middle of the night. They all have different roles, and all are important. Like the canes supporting the sweet peas, they are much stronger when they are tied together.

Over the years I have met a few people who were affected by sudden, severe mood swings, some of whom had been in long term care in hospital. These incidents of extreme mood change only happened to those individuals occasionally, sometimes a year or two apart, but in their worst form they could be life threatening. At the times when we were able to work closely with their psychiatrists, we might enable these volunteers to keep attending the garden. It was especially reassuring if their doctor could come to the garden that day and meet with the person, if we were concerned for their safety. This was hugely beneficial in working with someone so vulnerable. It was also very positive for the people concerned to know that they could live outside the hospital and still have immediate access to psychiatric support when they needed it.

HOW LONG SHOULD SUPPORT BE PROVIDED?

Back to the tomatoes.

Half-hardy plants will never be able to survive the winter alone, but if supported through those cold months, they will thrive and be productive during the warmer seasons. If a child is born with a disability or is involved in an accident and loses the use of a limb or one of their senses, then it is usually accepted that they might need some kind of support for the rest of their life. If they are given such support, they can often go on to live a fulfilled life. If someone is subjected to severe trauma as a child, caused by neglect or sexual, physical, or emotional abuse, to such an extent that it will affect them for the rest of their life, they are often expected to grow out of the need for support. People are often referred with medical notes saying, 'dependant personality', or even worse, 'attention seeking'. I feel those terms to be judgemental and damaging; they can follow people, in their case notes, for years. When you hear the person's story, it is no wonder they need some attention in that moment and quite possibly for the rest of their life.

This is not to say that people cannot recover and go on to lead fulfilling, independent lives. That should be our hope and goal for everyone. It simply means that support should not be limited to a time frame. Admitting to needing support should not be seen as a failure but as a brave attempt to live well in society. We all get buffeted by the trials of life and people who seem to have recovered their health might need support again if they go through a difficult patch.

Almost all mental health services are offered on a time-limited basis, with people having to leave the service when that time is up. This puts a huge strain on an individual and prevents them from having the courage to heal. If you have been traumatised at a young age, trust is understandably a big issue and it can take a long time to build it back up. If a Community Psychiatric Nurse or other mental health support worker is only offered for two months, or even two years, the work might only have just begun by the time they're scheduled to move on. You begin to get to know someone, begin to trust someone, begin to show some improvement, and before you know it they are saying, "I think we could drop your visits to fortnightly instead of weekly, don't you?" Soon they will stop all together. While these time scales might work for many, for severely traumatised individuals time limits on services can feel disastrous

This is not the fault of the support workers; they are just under too much pressure. The criteria for supporting people also often relates to domestic chores rather than emotional support. The questions frequently asked are:

- Can you shower by yourself?

- Can you use the washing machine?

- Can you shop for groceries?

The real question should be "*Do* you do these things?" Not "*Can* you?" I have known someone with a first-class engineering degree who could probably build you a washing machine from scratch but who struggled to actually put their own laundry into one. It wasn't that they didn't know how, they had just lost all motivation and energy. We also need to recognise that people who are very unwell are those most likely to be out of work and trying to live on state benefits. The assessment system can be brutal and degrading, and the amount of benefits that people are expected to live on is shockingly low. Many people spend more on a meal out than someone on benefits would have to last them a whole week. The 2019–2020 rate for universal credit is set at £317.82, which is less than £78 per week for an adult over twenty-five. You might get a rent payment on top of that, but you still have to pay for your utility bills, clothing, food and travel. If I go out for a meal it can easily be £20–£30, and that's not high-end dining by any means. A large part of a person's distress can be as simple as financial insecurity, born out of this impossibly small income. Even Monty Don, now national gardening guru of the BBC, who has suffered extremely poor mental health in the past, describes how "The whole experience of being unemployed is generally punitive. Your spirit sinks to the same level as your standard of living. I learnt to despise anyone who belittles the unemployed by accusing them of being work shy or lazy."[11]

It is always inspiring to see people's commitment to each other. It's easy to work in a garden in the summer when the weather is warm, the surroundings are beautiful and there is lots of food to take home at the end of the day. It is in the depths of winter that people showed their true commitment. In freezing weather in Scotland, with inches of snow on the ground, people will still come into the garden. Some come because they can't afford to heat their homes or face the loneliness, and others come to befriend them. They know how important it is to spend time in the garden, so they come to clear the driveway so that everyone can physically make it in. When the snow is bad enough to stop traffic, many volunteers and staff can have to walk a few miles to get there, especially if the buses aren't running. We light fires to keep people warm and bring soup, and someone will bake scones and bring them to share. People work really hard in difficult and trying conditions to help and support each other. These are often the same people that certain newspapers and right-leaning governments portray as cheats and benefits scroungers; the same people who, as Monty Don says, are branded work shy and lazy.

Half-hardy plants can flourish particularly well but only if protected when the cold weather comes. Similarly, many people can manage well for a time, but they do much better if they can get the support they need as soon as their mood begins to slip. Waiting months for a referral to be processed can put some people in real danger of slipping back into a worse state than before. When I started working in one garden, placements were time limited to two years and no re-entry for two years afterwards was allowed. Of course, some people just needed a bit of time to recover from whatever had happened to them, but more often than not, people had deeper, more long-standing problems. They would make great progress, then, a few months before the end of their placement, they would start to become anxious and stressed again. Two years to the day after they had left the garden because their time allowance was up, and they were back at the gate asking for a new placement and all the gains had been lost – the classic 'revolving door' effect, which we will explore in Chapter 12. People need to be allowed as much time as it takes to recover. Most people recover within a two-year period, some more quickly. But for people who have deeply rooted trauma, recovery can't, and should not be, time-limited.

Cost factors are often thrown up as the reason for time-limited services. However, the cost of supporting someone in a garden (as a day service) is minimal compared to keeping someone in a psychiatric hospital.

> The cost of psychiatric care in a hospital … is estimated at approximately £2,900 per month *[2007 source]*.
> *www.networks.nhs.uk*[12]

Even if this figure is more than a decade ago already, a fraction of that amount per person could pay for a well-funded, professionally staffed mental health gardening service. It would only need to keep a few people out of hospital to pay for itself. Beyond the financial benefits, there are huge bonuses for the individual and the community; people stay healthier, are more productive, learn a skill, and avoid being institutionalised and stigmatised.

A tell-tale comment I have heard many times from individuals who have been hospitalised was that people seldom visit you in a psychiatric hospital. The wards are not festooned with gifts and flowers, and there are rarely any children. While it is true that many psychiatric hospitals have improved greatly, it should be seen as immensely cost-effective and much more positive to provide support via community gardens and other community-based mental health projects, rather than secluding people in hospitals if it can be avoided.

SUPPORTING THE STAFF

In some of the gardens I worked in, particularly if they were specifically for people experiencing mental health problems, there was a professional staff team who needed support too. In that kind of set up, everyone in the garden does – the volunteers, the core staff, the office staff, the manager, and even the public.

Core staff cannot work successfully with trauma if they themselves do not feel supported. People often go into this kind of work thinking it is about helping other people change their behaviour, and it can be quite a shock for them to realise how much time they will have to spend looking at, and changing, their own behaviour. This kind of work can be emotionally charged, difficult, and soul-searching, and needs to be supported openly. For example, a new volunteer might come on site and, through nobody's fault, they don't get on with a particular member of staff. Sometimes their difficulty is as simple as a family resemblance, but at other times it can be much more complicated. That volunteer needs the staff support as much as any other, so it's a situation that needs to be worked through.

In this model of co-working, the team all are on an equal footing, albeit with different roles and responsibilities. Each member of the team knows what his or her responsibilities are; these are worked out carefully together, so that the best use is made of everyone's skill. Allowing longer staff team meetings is never a waste of time. In a therapeutic garden, I found it really valuable to meet up to three times a day, if only for a quick fifteen-minute planning session in the morning, a roll call and check in at midday, and a quick debrief at the end of the day. Because you are meeting several times a day and talking together often, the team tends to develop a kind of shorthand; because everyone knows the context, you don't have to keep getting people up to speed. If, very occasionally, something serious happens to someone during the day, you might feel the need to retire to a coffee shop after work until everyone feels happy to go home. This last check-in is the most important: ensuring that no-one is leaving the garden worried about something troubling they have said or heard and not shared. It's also important to have regular staff training days. Each member of staff can be encouraged to bring a topic to share, either because they need to learn about it from the rest of the team, or because they have learnt something new and want to share it. The topics people might bring to these meetings might vary enormously: from mind mapping tools, which will help with planning, to feedback on a course about trauma; from a catch up on the garden features being created, to a breakdown on budget spending.

SUPPORTING THE MANAGER

On one particular training day, I set out large sheets of paper and coloured crayons and asked the team to draw their ideal manager. The image that sticks in my mind was of a figure lying on a deck chair under an umbrella on a tropical island, drinking a long cold drink, surrounded by clear skies and blue sea. I was a bit flummoxed and asked the artist if she wanted me to go on holiday, but she said no. What did she want then? She said she wanted her manager to be calm. It was an insightful moment.

When you are managing a substantial mental health service, there are always at least three crises a day, and it is very easy to get sucked into them and to feel your own stress levels rising. It was great feedback, which I probably would never have got if I hadn't made time for such a visually creative exercise. The image has stayed with me, whereas her words might not have. Other members of the team often acted as something of a barometer and would periodically say things like: "You can take your finger off the panic button now." I felt looked after by those team members who were so honest and direct with me. As a manager, the most helpful support you can get is from your team. The salaries for these kind of jobs are usually relatively low, even though staff often come highly qualified, with degrees or diplomas in some kind of environmental studies, as well as some qualification or experience in mental health. Working conditions can also be fairly primitive. No one accepts this kind job for money or prestige, and they are usually deeply committed people, many of whom have had their own tangles with depression, anxiety and trauma, and are passionate about the healing powers of working in a garden.

ORGANISATIONAL SUPPORT

In any expansive welfare organisation, there is a great responsibility to make sure that every project is operating safely and ethically. How do you ensure that everyone is working to the required standard? Do you give guidelines for every occasion? How cumbersome that would be, even if it were possible. Do you endlessly ask for audits on health and safety, policy adherence and so forth, and end up using valuable time to complete them? How do you safeguard each individual? It's truly a dilemma.

I believe the process starts with how you approach interviewing candidates. In the first big garden I worked in, which was a residential unit for children, prospective candidates were required to come for a 24-hour visit with an overnight stay. When I became responsible for hiring staff for a garden or day service, I would invite people to come for an informal pre-interview visit and work with us for the day, followed by a full-day 'interview' procedure. This involved them leading a group teaching session on a simple horticultural task, before joining all the volunteers for a discussion group and lunch. Finally, there was a formal interview with two staff members and a volunteer. Volunteer feedback was included in our assessment of candidates. A formal interview alone only lets you see how well people perform in a formal setting and can be very misleading.

In their book *The Tidal Model*[13], Phil and Poppy Barker outline their person-centred recovery approach to mental health, which emphasises helping people to reclaim their personal story, to recover their own voice, and subsequently to regain control over their own lives. The authors talk about 'commitments not commandments' for staff. If you work with a set of rules to cover every eventuality, you have to write down a commandment for every conceivable scenario someone might encounter, and then you monitor their adherence to them. The task would be enormous. For example, one such rule I found impossible to adhere to in every situation was that members of staff should not give their mobile phone numbers to volunteers. I understand why that rule was made. It was not considered safe or appropriate, for many reasons, for staff to have personal relationships with volunteers that included having one-to-one conversations on private phones outside of garden hours. This, among other considerations, can set up a false sense of how available staff might be in an emergency out of working hours. At that time, I also had a leading role in two different voluntary projects in the town where I live. My mobile number was freely available on their websites and notices. A few volunteers became involved in those projects which were widely publicised and so of course had access to my mobile number. They used it when appropriate and never otherwise, so no problem arose. In that situation I had to make a judgement to break the rules and allow people from the garden to contact me about these other projects, using my personal mobile. To do anything else would have been to stigmatise them. Everyone involved seemed to completely understand their commitment to my right to privacy.

Alternatively, you can teach people a philosophy, some principles of practice, and ask them to commit to it. With this method, you teach staff how to use their own judgement wisely, adhering to the values they have learnt. On occasions when the situation seems to have arisen outside of all the guidelines and no supervisory person is available, staff have to make their own decisions and their own risk assessment of the situation. This has the benefit of covering unpredictable scenarios, which arise more often than you might think, but demands a thorough training and understanding of the philosophy of the company and the integrity of the people within it.

It can be complex. I was at a conference once where the speaker, a mental health nurse, related a story from her own experience. With permission, she had taken a small group of people from the hospital where she worked for a walk in the countryside. When they were some way from the hospital, the day became much warmer than expected, and one of the women really needed a cold drink and to use the toilet. The woman was beginning to get quite distressed when the nurse realised they were only a few minutes away from her own cottage. Thinking it to be the kindest course of action, she took the group to her home, allowed them to use the facilities, gave them all a drink, let them have a wee rest to cool, then they all walked back to the hospital. She was severely reprimanded for her actions, i.e. taking patients into her own home. The nurse's behaviour stepped outside the accepted professional boundaries for sure, but she was faced with an unexpected situation where someone in her care was distressed. She made a judgement based on compassion. While realising those rules are put in place to protect everyone sometimes it can be hard to know the best course of action.

It is a bit like the law on health and safety in the workplace, the Health and Safety at Work Act of 1974. It started out with a long list of rules, but then incidents kept cropping up that weren't covered by it. This made it difficult to settle lawsuits and easy for employers to wriggle out of responsibility – if the incident hadn't been foreseen, then they hadn't broken any rules. The law was then changed. Although there are guidelines, the main thrust of the act is that employers must take 'every reasonable precaution' to keep their employees safe. They have to accept the intention of the law and use their own judgement.

All these different structures of support – legal, financial, medical, psychiatric, horticultural, and interpersonal or informal – work better if coordinated and put in place with sensitivity, compassion, flexibility, and transparency. They need to be based in practical, lived experience. This way, everyone and everything has a far better chance of thriving and flourishing.

KEY POINTS
Support and protection

- Sometimes, just knowing that someone else can see your distress is enough.

- It seldom takes one magic spell to shift a low mood; instead, a collection of small, different approaches can gradually make a difference.

- The scars from emotional trauma can inflict such damage that, just as with physical conditions, someone might need support for most of their life. People can learn to manage their emotional wounds better but cannot necessarily 'grow out of them'.

- With the right support, people can flourish and live fulfilling and productive lives.

- Meaningful involvement takes a lot of time, expertise and energy.

- Encourage honest feedback, even if it's critical.

- A committed team works better than one that simply follows all the rules.

CHAPTER 10

PESTS, DISEASES, DISORDERS

"To maintain my sanity, I need at least one full day a week in the garden. It works better than any pills, better than any medicine. Earth heals!"

Monty Don[14]

The key principles of organic growth are to provide the best conditions for health. However, we are working in the unpredictable realm of nature. Despite our best efforts, plants can fail to thrive. Some are minor setbacks, which are easily overcome. For example, seedlings might get stretched and spindly because they are overcrowded and are not getting enough light and space. This can easily be solved by 'pricking out'. Seeds are sown into seed compost, which has an open texture and allows for drainage, but it does not typically contain much in the way of nutrients. When the seedlings begin to fill the container they need to be transplanted, very carefully, to give them more space into a more nutrient-rich compost.

SO WHAT CAN GO WRONG?

Pests are insects or animals which live off, weaken or destroy your plants. Greenhouses are notoriously prone to infestation from aphids – prolific, tiny insects which can suck the life out of your tomato plants. There are some organic sprays you can use, such as basic soapy water, but usually the best solution is to bring in some parasitic wasps. These will happily feast on the

aphids and sort that out for you. You can also plant companion plants which attract the predators you want. For example,
Limnanthes, commonly called the poached egg plant because
it looks exactly like one, will attract hover flies which will help
keep down aphid numbers down. Similarly, outdoors, some
plants such as nasturtiums, marigolds and chives will deter
pests you don't want and attract another friend, the ladybird,
and with luck you can let nature take its course.
These plants look pretty and usually they have
a strong smell. They will support one another in
their life cycles.

It's important to be flexible. If one of your children decides
to become a vegetarian, you usually don't give the rest of your
kids sausage, peas and chips and just take the sausage off the
vegetarian's plate. This would result in a completely unbalanced
diet. Instead, you would have to approach his diet with the aim
of making sure he has the correct amount of protein, among
other nutrients. Using the same analogy of childrearing, if you
decide you want to avoid overusing chemicals and drugs such
as antibiotics on your children, then you have to make sure
they have a healthy diet, get plenty of exercise, practise good
hygiene and get enough rest. In organic gardening, you can't
use chemicals to protect a crop but you can use barriers like
nets and fleece to keep pests at bay. There are many other natural ways to deal with problems, including good nutrition and
cultivation – pests seem less likely to attack strong plants.

Disorders and diseases can occur in plants because of min-
eral deficiencies, growing conditions, lack of nutrients, viruses,
infections and mutations. These can often be prevented by the
smart use of garden compost and animal manure – my current
favourite is donkey poo produced in abundance by the delight-
ful and handsome Monty – to return nutrients to the soil, and

good housekeeping to clean out any infections in green houses or pots for old plant debris. Not all disorders are unwanted. For example, variegated privet is prized for its bright colours. Instead of being dark green, it has two colours, yellow and light green. Although they are not as tough as the green privet (because variegation is most commonly a mutation in the plant, which weakens it), they are much more beautiful. It can cheer up a dull winter's day to see their golden glow in the garden.

CULTIVATION

Even the healthiest of plants will suffer damage when subjected to stressful conditions such as drought, high winds, severe frosts, or vandalism. With foresight, the effects of these can be avoided; as discussed in previous chapters, mulching, careful watering, staking and protection all help.

Sometimes, a fruit tree will bear so much fruit that you might decide to remove some of it before it reaches maturity. This is to help the tree produce good-sized, edible fruit. If you leave all the apples to keep growing in a heavy crop, you are likely to get lots and lots of very hard small fruit. If you remove every other apple when they are still small early in the season, the ones you leave will grow on to be bigger, juicier fruit. You might also have to add supports to the laden boughs during the fruiting season, in case the weight makes the bough break.

PRUNING

Pruning the garden is an on-going business, as plants need to be pruned at different times. The golden rule of thumb among gardeners is to cut away the four Ds: dead, diseased, dying, damaged. That done, you might want to prune for a specific desired shape, or for ease of collecting the fruit.

Damaged growth needs to be removed. If you need to prune back the damaged limb of an apple tree to remove a problem growth, it's unlikely you'll get a great crop of apples that year. It might take two to three years, or maybe even more, for the tree to recover, depending on how severe the damage is. The tree might always need some extra support if, for example, a large bough has been broken and the tree has become unbalanced. However, in time you will get a much happier tree with more bountiful fruit, so the pruning, feeding and tending are well worth the effort.

Sometimes, you might begin to give up hope and feel that all your work has been in vain, as the plant does not seem to be recovering. This can be very disheartening, and it is sometimes difficult to remain hopeful, especially if the plant needs a lot of attention. However, there's a sense in which all things in nature 'want to get well'. Underneath the surface, changes are occurring unnoticed; if you're patient, the plant will sometimes recover by itself. It may never be as fruitful as a plant that has always been healthy, but it will often recover sufficiently to give a good crop.

If only we could prune our lives as easily as we do an apple tree. I suspect few of us find it easy to regularly de-clutter our homes, give up habits that deplete our energy or make us ill, and learn to stay away from negative influences. For many people, getting rid of belongings that they have held onto for many years is hugely difficult, even when it's obvious that it's making their home a hazardous, uncomfortable place to be. What looks like clutter to other people, can be like a nest for the individual; a well-known safe place to hide in, the cradle of their identity.

Terry worked as a silversmith making jewellery, a highly-skilled job which demanded unique expertise. There were few people who could do the kind of work he did. He kept meticulous records and notes of all the projects he worked on and he had a large collection of reference books. As his work became more demanding and stressful, he began to get unwell and eventually had to give up the work that was his lifetime achievement. Terry lived in a very small flat so there was limited space when he took home all his precious notes and files – he considered these a record of his whole working life and he felt defined by them. As his room grew more cluttered, the space became as stressful as his employment situation. He lived like this for many years, growing increasingly upset. He needed these boxes of files to remind him that he was a skilled and valued person, but they were preventing him from creating a comfortable, functional home. Eventually, once he was certain he would never return to his old line of work, he recognised that they were holding him back from moving on to a new occupation.

Conversations with Terry went a bit like this:

"If I throw away all my old newspaper articles about my work, will I start to forget who I really am?"

"If I get rid of my old files will people forget that I was once very competent?"

"I need to sort out all this 'stuff' and clear most of it out because it's driving me mad and I need to move on somehow."

"But if I throw out all my…" and so on. It became cyclical.

We were getting nowhere and he was becoming ever more distressed. He wasn't ready to throw it all out, but he didn't have the space to sort through it and couldn't go on living with it. Although it served to remind him of what he had achieved, it also saddened him with what he felt he had lost. And his living space was a mess.

We worked together to identify a storage space he could use temporarily – a friend's garage. It had to be an interim solution because it would get very damp in winter. It was somewhere he could store the boxes and go through them to decide what could be destroyed or given away and what really needed to be kept. He gladly accepted this offer. It gave him some breathing space and meant he could at least get on with sorting out his home without the clutter of his precious files. He managed to gather his numerous boxes, which almost filled the garage, and the owner reminded him that they would not overwinter well and that he had six months to sort through them.

After a few months, his home situation and mood were much improved; he began to recover his health and left the garden. He never did return to sort through his boxes, despite several reminders that the boxes was getting damp. A few years later, when the friend really needed the space, she tried in vain to contact him again. When his paperwork was inspected, it had been completely ruined by the damp. We had news from his friends that he was well and thriving, so he was contacted one final time to let him know the situation, saying that if the friend didn't hear from him she would dispose of the boxes. There was still no response. It seemed that time had helped him separate from his past and that he no longer needed his boxes of memories.

As with a precious plant, 'pruning' in someone's life should always be approached with great caution. 'De-cluttering' can leave the person feeling very exposed and vulnerable. What needs to be disposed of might seem obvious to an outsider but that ignores the emotional attachment a person might have to a set of objects or to another person, or even to a habitual behaviour.

PRE-EXISTING CONDITIONS

Some people coming to a garden have a pre-existing condition, such as dyslexia, hearing and sight impairments, or epilepsy, which have had a serious impact on their mental health.

These conditions, in themselves, are not mental health problems. However, mistreatment and poor management of these and other conditions can certainly cause them to develop into mental health issues, especially if people have been repeatedly unsupported, misunderstood and bullied because of their condition. I have met many wonderful artists who were dyslexic, who had been made to feel vulnerable because their condition had not been met with understanding. These people challenged the way we taught and the way we worked, and they made us better at how we communicated with everyone. It was a real gift to the garden when we had a member of staff who had a condition such as dyslexia and was not distressed by it. They were able to give witness to the fact that it was not the dyslexia that was the issue, but the way it had been handled in people's lives. It's a bit like giving an azalea plant to someone who doesn't know anything about their specific needs. It can be a beautiful healthy specimen when given an acid soil, but if it is planted under a wall which has been leaching lime into the soil, making it very alkaline, it will not thrive. In this case, there is nothing wrong with the plant itself, it just hasn't been given the right growing conditions. If you dig it up and transplant it into some acid soil, it will usually regain its vigour.

ACQUIRED DISABILITY

Some people would come to the garden having had a breakdown in their mental health following an accident or illness that has resulted in a certain loss of function. While the disability was often very specific, and may not have appeared severe to an outsider, you have to consider the loss in the context of that person's life, to get a true sense of its impact.

> George, a man in his late forties, came to the garden having lost his job after he developed arthritis of the knees. He could walk fairly well and on first impression seemed fit and strong. It was only on finding out that he used to be a football coach that the extent of his depression and his feeling of loss began to make sense. His job was his whole life; his identity. It provided him with his peer group, his status in society, and with proper pride in what he was doing. It is not necessarily a disaster to lose a job, but this man lost his career as well, which is a completely different thing. He had been a football coach for nearly twenty years and was not trained to do anything else. More importantly, he did not want to do anything else. His sadness was exacerbated by his inability to find another job. Unsurprisingly, he didn't present very well at interviews because he had no experience or enthusiasm for the work on offer.

Within six months, his finances were in ruins and he could no longer pay the mortgage. His personality seemed to have changed completely and his marriage was in trouble. George lost his job, his career, his status, his confidence, his home, and his wife, in just over a year.

It took a few years of being in the garden and being allowed to mourn that loss before he began to remember that he did have other skills and that he could still be successful doing other things. He became a very good gardener and handyman in time, and eventually left when he got a job doing just that in a care home for the elderly.

Compared to some people, this man was relatively lucky. He came with serious mental health issues, but in the past he had possessed all the skills required to live well in society. He had a great work ethic, was punctual, understood different levels of responsibility, and was able to take responsibility for his own work. He was good at making relationships and got on well with his colleagues; he knew how to manage personal and household finances; he could feed and look after himself, and manage a home. He didn't have to learn all these things from scratch: he just had to remember them. Bereavement, inappropriate promotion (where a new role puts unmanageable stress on a worker who has previously been very competent at their work), general work stresses, divorce, and homelessness can have a similar affect. All contain elements of loss: loss of confidence, loss of a sense of self, and loss of status.

Given the right conditions to heal, people can and do go on to begin a new career and live successfully.

PEOPLE AFFECTED BY TRAUMA SINCE EARLY CHILDHOOD

People who have never learnt important life skills due to bad parenting, or a lack of parenting, and childhood traumas can experience different, more lasting challenges. Their childhood might have included physical, mental or sexual abuse (or a toxic combination of these), neglect and bullying, and being brought up in serial institutions, with all the consequent effects described in Chapter 10.

These people may never have had the opportunity to make friends easily, if at all. They may never have had the confidence to try new things, go to new places, or apply for jobs. This is a different challenge altogether. As outlined before, the old habits that worked for a time to help a frightened child feel safe in an unhealthy environment do not usually work to launch a person into the adult world. Those habits need to be unpicked and new skills learnt that will allow the person to live a meaningful and fulfilled adult life. This should certainly include appropriate and rewarding work, where possible, forging healthy relationships and generally learning to survive in the outside world.

Imagine you were born in a time when people believed that the earth was flat, when all maps were made according to that belief. Then along came someone who said, "No, the world is round", and produced a globe. They took you up a high hill where you could see the surface of the earth curving away from you and you began to understand that it must be true. However, you didn't know how to read the contours of a globe and all the continents were a different shape. The whole world had a different focus. You were told you would not fall off if you kept walking, but you had believed this all of your life and avoided the 'edges'.

It must have been terrifying for people to begin to take on the enormity of that change in perspective. When suddenly you find the route map you have been using all your life is flawed, you are left in a place with no map at all. Even when you are given a new map, it can seem as if it's written in a foreign language that you still have to learn.

It takes a while to get past the confusion and fear of the unknown, to begin to learn to work with the new maps. For many people, a change like this feels as if the place they are standing on is crumbling and their only escape is to walk across a deep chasm to a new place. But they can't actually see the bridge they are being asked to cross. When they touch it, it feels rickety and unsafe and gives them a tremendous fear of falling. They have no idea what is on the other side.

When this happened with someone in the garden, I could only try to reassure them that we had crossed the bridge many times with others before them, and that we knew from experience that the place on the other side was healthier and happier than the place they were in now. We also had to acknowledge that it could be a harrowing bridge to cross, but that we were willing to walk over it with them. Once you understand this kind of flat earth thinking, i.e. when people are working from a very different set of rules and beliefs, then unusual or seemingly strange behaviour on their part begins to make more sense.

The garden and nature itself, at first, can offer a safe relationship when trusting other people feels too difficult. The beauty of a big garden community is that there are always, in my experience, kind, compassionate people to take a new person under their wing, to teach them skills, and gradually win their trust and build their confidence. Animals help, too. Many gardens employ a cat to stop the mice from eating all the seeds. Many a cat earns his keep as a brilliant friend and support to everyone. It's also common to have regular visits from various lovable docile dogs that everyone enjoys cuddling.

As we saw in 'emotional weeding', the effects of childhood abuse and trauma are manifold and complicated. A few essential points are worth mentioning again here.

Gabor Mate[15] is a leading expert on addiction – addiction to work, exercise, overeating, dieting, drinking, smoking, gambling, gaming, drug and alcohol dependence, and, in his own case, addiction to buying music recordings. He believes that people's behaviour makes sense when you understand their story. They may have a history of neglect, sexual, emotional or physical abuse, or they might have the sense of nothingness that comes from the daily drip of being ignored, of being bullied, or of grieving for a loved one, a home, limb, job, or loss of physical health. I experienced many instances when I felt this to be true; when someone's behaviour seemed completely illogical at first, but gradually, as I came to know their story, it began to make sense.

Telling your story can be anything but straightforward, as often we don't understand it ourselves. Sometimes people tell their story nonverbally: by hurting themselves, isolating themselves, neglecting to care for themselves, not eating and/or gorging on food, or overworking. They try to be perfect so as not to stand out; you become visible when you make mistakes.

Last spring, I grew a number of tomato plants from seed. They were all growing well so I kept three for myself in my small greenhouse and planted six in the polytunnel in a community garden where I work. The ones in my greenhouse quickly grew and bore masses of flowers and fruit, but the ones in the community garden did nothing at all for several weeks and some of them began to look quite discoloured.

I tried various things. I gave them a good compost mulch, I fed them with a tomato feed, I checked they were not being attacked by pests. For several weeks they languished and I couldn't figure out what was wrong.

One day, I noticed there were some people from the shop next to the garden standing outside having a smoke. It suddenly hit me that in all probability, when we weren't there and it was raining, people would shelter in the polytunnel to smoke and that it was probably tobacco mosaic virus that was infecting the tomatoes.

I had to live with those plants for quite a while and observe them carefully to understand which external factors were affecting them, and I only found out by accident at that.

The Tidal Model[16] describes "the power of the pen". People need to be allowed to tell their story in their own words, in their own language, and not have it paraphrased or edited. It doesn't matter if you fully understand it so long as the person telling it does. By giving people the power to write their own notes which can be added to the minutes of the meeting, or by allowing them time to edit the ones you have written, you can make a big difference to the veracity of what is captured. This can also even out the perceived balance of power between staff and volunteers, or doctors and patients.

Too frequently, this doesn't happen in practice. When people are attending medical and mental health services, they are usually interviewed, rather than engaged in a conversation.

A member of staff takes notes, which are their interpretation of what has been said, and so the document becomes the product of both people's life stories. The person telling their story is not usually given a copy of the notes. He or she does not get to read it or sign it. These written records of interviews can follow an individual for years, a lifetime even, and they can affect the way future services respond to that individual.

EMPATHY OR EXPERTISE

Everyone should be allowed to tell their story. While many people with trauma in their background want to do it, indeed are often driven to do it, they also describe it as humiliating, exhausting, sad, and eventually, with many repetitions, it can even become boring (which is actually usually seen as a good sign as all the emotion has been leached out of it). Hopefully in time, people move on from talking about what has happened to them in the past and will recover some degree of health and the ability to flourish.

Sometimes, however, I feel that an individual's need to have me understand exactly what they are feeling becomes so all-consuming that it might actually be doing them harm. It can take them years of constantly revisiting tragic life events. In their attempts to explain, they are continually re-traumatising themselves and causing themselves great distress. Knowing that I can never truly understand what they are feeling because, thankfully, I have never had to endure similar experiences, I will sometimes tell them about my car. Let me explain.

When I was younger, our car used to break down regularly, probably because we were not well off and usually bought old bangers. I know very little about car mechanics. I had two choices when my car broke down. I could visit a neighbour whose car was always breaking down, in the knowledge that he would understand exactly how I was feeling and be able to empathise with my predicament, but probably wouldn't be able to sort it out. Or I could go and visit the neighbour whose car never seemed to break down. He would probably not be able to understand how I was feeling but if I was prepared to learn from him, I might be able to understand what he did to look after and maintain his car in order to keep it running smoothly. This would involve some study, regular allocation of time and effort, and it would not be a quick fix. If I had been really lucky, I might have had a neighbour who, in the past, had experienced cars that kept breaking down, but had succeeded in learning how to run her car smoothly. In her, I would have found both empathy and helpful know-how.

DEPRESSION

Sometimes self-help groups can offer this kind of support; their combination of empathy, understanding and skill-sharing is invaluable.

Depression Alliance[17], one of the groups I worked with regularly, came up with the expression 'get out of your head and into your life'. Doing, not thinking, can really help people move on. Working in a garden is both physically and mentally challenging. It absorbs the attention and so it can give people a rest from the awful thoughts and feelings that may be plaguing them. They can get back to being 'nicely tired' rather than worried and worn out.

As described in the wonderful carton book by Matthew Johnstone, *I Had a Black Dog*[18], depression hates physical activity and the best way to beat it is to get active or to encourage someone suffering from it to get active.

CRISIS HUNTING

I was once given a T-shirt that said:

> Any idiot can cope with a crisis, it's the day to day living that
> wears you out.

It was in response to a discussion about what is known as 'crisis hunting'.[19] It can happen to anyone who has to live with a high level of anxiety for a long period of time. I once had to work with a very unpredictable group who, without warning, could get very angry: something I found particularly challenging.

I got so used to being on high alert with lots of adrenaline pumping through my system that after I had left that group and was working elsewhere, I was still stuck in that mode and constantly looking for problems, even beginning to create them, because of my hyper-vigilance and prickliness. It took quite a few comments like,

> "Why is this bothering you so much, it really doesn't matter
> does it?"

> "Are you sure this is worth getting so upset about?"

> "Has someone hit your panic button?"

before I realised what was happening. I was so used to living in a high-adrenalin state that even though things had got much better, I didn't want to let my guard down. It had become a habit, so living without that rush felt a bit flat and empty, even though I knew it was caused by, and generated, distress. I had become a crisis junkie. It's quite hard to explain if you have never experienced it but the experience is well-documented.

I was so used to too much adrenalin coursing through my system that I had to painstakingly teach myself to adjust to a calmer state of being. I had to step back before I reacted and try to look for the amicable way out of disputes rather than immediately switching into battle mode. I also had to learn to recognise calmness as a feeling of being peaceful and at ease, rather than a sense of being flat and uncomfortable.

The distress I went through then was minor and short lived in comparison to that of many of our volunteers. I was often told of situations in which people lived in fear of abuse, humiliation, violence and neglect, or even literally in fear of their lives. This may have gone on for many years, until they were old enough or sufficiently supported by someone, to break away from the situation.

That constant habit of hyper-vigilance and high alert is very difficult to shake. Learning to live with the ordinary is much harder than it seems

KEY POINTS
Pests, diseases, disorders

- We all thrive in different growing conditions. It takes time to find out what those are for different individuals.

- Loss has to be seen in the context of someone's life. Comparisons are not useful.

- The confidence gained through a newly learnt skill spills over into other areas of a person's life.

- The best support offers empathy and teaches new skills.

- Doing, not thinking, is often the best way to help people out of depression.

- To build up 'emotional muscle' you have to exercise regularly even when it hurts, i.e. if you are feeling scared and anxious, it is OK to ask for help even if you find that difficult to do.

- Panic attacks are terrifying, but with the right help and understanding, they can quickly be brought under control.

- People want to be able to give something back to society as well as to receive help. Sometimes, using your own experiences to help others can make something good come out of something distressing.

CHAPTER 11

HARVESTING

The harvest is the fruit – the fruit of the plant and of the gardener's hard work, care, and good husbandry. At last there is something to taste, to eat, and to enjoy, which will also carry the seed forward. It happens in different cycles for different plants. Whereas radishes will be ready in six weeks, Brussels sprouts take the whole season, and a newly planted apple tree might take several years before it yields fruit.

Harvests can be unpredictable. You can't control the weather and a late frost might kill all the blossom on an apple tree, meaning no fruit will appear that year. Despite this, the plant itself will not be affected but will go on growing and storing energy until next year when it might have a bumper crop.

Harvest festivals are heavy with symbolism for a reason. They remind us of the earth's precious bounty and ability to renew itself. But they also encourage us to reflect on how fragile the earth can be, and how we shouldn't take it for granted.

When you talk about harvest time, people usually think of late autumn when the apples are picked or indeed of those harvest festivals popular in churches and schools, usually in late September or early October. Many vegetables and fruit are ready for harvest in late autumn, such as potatoes, apples, pears and turnips. However, only an inexperienced gardener would harvest once a year. The real skill is in having something ready to eat the whole year round. Sow little and often is the smart gardener's motto, so that you can have salads ready the whole year round, then other produce in succession. Sprouting broccoli, leeks and kale emerge in the cold months at the beginning of the year when nothing else grows. All the soft fruits, plums, tomatoes, cucumber, peas and beans come during the summer. Then potatoes, carrots and parsnips can be lifted in the autumn and stored for the winter months, as can some of the apples and pears which can be dried for you to eat through the winter.

It's a lovely feeling to put food into storage against the 'hungry gap', the term gardeners use for the period between the end of winter and the arrival of the first spring vegetables, when little grows and nothing produces crops. Similarly, it's good to freeze some raspberries to have at Christmas. Some flowers, like sweet peas, need to be constantly cut to keep them producing: the more you cut the more you get. Other flowers can be dried and pressed to give you the pleasure of their beauty all the year round like lavender, which can be dried and put to many different uses, including tucking some under your pillow to help you sleep.

Harvesting in the garden is always a great feeling, whether it's wandering round the garden, picking raspberries and popping them into your mouth, collecting a handful of mangetout peas to chomp on as you go, or pulling a ripe plum off a branch and eating it, warm and sun-kissed straight from the tree. Then, at the end of the week, everyone goes home with a rewarding bag of freshly picked fruit and veg, the best the earth has to offer. For someone who has never grown anything before, and who is also living on a very small budget, it's little short of a miracle.

From time to time, people who have left come back for a visit and tell you how they have been getting on. Many go on to gardening careers, some go back to their old line of work, either paid or in a voluntary way, and others do something completely different. It is always great to see people make enough progress to get back out there and try to make a better life for themselves, sometimes returning with new partners and children, stories to tell, and an enthusiasm for life. Those who come back to work as staff in a therapeutic garden have something really special to offer current volunteers. They are able to say with total honesty, "I know how you are feeling because I was there once. It will get better."

> The school for emotionally distressed children where I worked for ten years was one of the most expensive in the UK. The headmaster was invited to give a talk on its unorthodox ways of working (unusual for the 1970s that is). At question time, a member of the audience asked if it was worth the amount of money it cost to run. Did the headmaster have any figures of positive outcomes in later life to justify the expense?
>
> He replied that he didn't have to justify it. The boys at the school had been damaged by a society that had failed to protect and look after them, and they deserved the best possible upbringing and care that could be provided, no matter what the outcome was.

As with the garden's harvest, people don't get better in a single day. There will be good days and bad. Things fluctuate on a day-to-day basis, little achievements accumulate along the way, as do resources, strength and resilience. Sometimes there are real landmarks and sometimes there are false ones. For people who become anxious in groups, one of their myriad landmarks might be managing to eat in public – an activity that can make you feel conspicuous if you get it wrong. Other landmarks might involve staying in the room for the first time during a meeting, offering to make the tea for everyone at break time or showing someone how to do something. It can be as simple as someone lifting their eyes from the floor to look at you, however briefly, when they are talking to you, and, importantly, asking for help. These are the steps that gradually enable people to get their life back.

Some people say that they will try out the suggestions for improving their health – going out for a walk every day, stopping drinking coffee, joining a yoga class – once they are feeling better. While I can see the reasoning behind this, it doesn't work. It's like telling the physio that you will do the exercises when your back stops being sore. You have to start building emotional muscle when it is still hurting. This is hard and the results are not very noticeable at first. As with physiotherapy, it might actually feel worse before it gets better. But gradually, doing the exercises pays off and you begin to feel the results. It may not mean all your problems have gone away, but they might be more manageable and you might get closer to leading the life you want.

One common result of being very anxious is that people experience panic attacks.[20] During such an attack, which can happen anywhere, there is a sudden sense of extreme anxiety[21] and fear – a dread that something unsurvivable is going to happen. Symptoms of a panic attack include a pounding heart, feeling dizzy, feeling as though you are going to pass out, being short of breath and having chest pains, sweating, shaking, and feeling sick. Of course, these conditions do resemble that of a heart attack and this needs to be ruled out by a doctor before the person is diagnosed with having panic attacks.

All of these feelings of panic are a natural response to danger, where the body is put into "fight or flight" mode. When you are faced with danger, your body thinks you can either stay and fight it or run away as fast as you can. Imagine being a caveperson, standing in the wild, facing a large and dangerous animal. To help you cope with this, your body floods you with adrenalin which causes all the above symptoms. However, in physical terms we have by and large moved on from being attacked by wild animals. What often frightens people who are anxious is social embarrassment. In this situation, the flight or fight response has grown way out of proportion. Once triggered, the fear of having a panic attack is often enough to trigger another one.

People tend to experience one or two panic attacks in their lifetime, but for some this leads to more frequent attacks. In an extreme case, this fear can cause an individual to withdraw from any situation that might make them anxious, and so their life becomes quite socially restrictive. Sadly, this behaviour only reinforces their thinking that shops, cinemas, restaurants and the like are dangerous places, and so begins a downward spiral. What seems to help most with managing panic attacks is for the individual to learn as much as possible about what causes them. This helps them grasp techniques for managing them. There are many excellent books and websites which can help with this. They include learning to control your thinking, your breathing and your fear.

I have met several people with a history of severe mental health problems who happened to be very good public speakers. They were, in general terms, still quite unwell, but on occasion they could put that aside and give a speech to a hundred people. This was all the more impressive and valuable because of their lived experience. On stage, they appeared to be completely in control and managed the situation beautifully. People in the audience would be full of praise for them. Then once out of the public eye they would be completely exhausted; it would often take them at least a week to regain some equilibrium. I hasten to say that giving the speech was always the individual's choice and sometimes it was made against advice because others were afraid it would be too draining for them.

Jerry, in particular, seemed to get much more anxious after he had done some public speaking (which he was very good at and really wanted to do). So much so that I questioned whether it was worth it for him. He eventually explained to me that it wasn't the public speaking that was hard; he had been used to giving speeches for many years. It was the praise afterwards. He felt that if people thought he could manage to do that, then there couldn't be that much wrong with him, rendering him a fraud. People often believe that the harvest only comes at the end of the season and that anything achieved earlier is some kind of trickery.

It's important to appreciate the skills that you have, like being able to give a talk. These skills don't necessarily go away because you are anxious or depressed, just as you don't forget how to drive or use the toaster. In a therapeutic garden, one of the really useful harvests that people gleaned from their own illness was developing and presenting educational talks and displays around mental health. This could even take the form of showing a visitor round – a great opportunity to influence people's understanding of mental health and the value of a therapeutic garden. Community gardens are always getting requests for visits. Volunteers can get involved in developing presentations for these groups, and with hosting visits, a perfect opportunity to spread the word about the power of working in a garden.

This can be an especially empowering opportunity for people to use their painful experiences to inform others' understanding of mental health problems. They are best placed to explain how poor mental health can affect people's lives, and most importantly how they can affect anyone of any walk of life. This process of illuminating others can go a long way towards helping individuals feel better about themselves. It can be seen as a way of giving back to society – a thank you for the help they themselves have received and a way of making things better for others.

Those who get involved with developing educational material on mental health always seem to progress faster in their own understanding of their own road to recovery. You have to learn to look at your own situation from a distance and develop what is described as the 'observing self' – trying to use the rational part of your brain to observe your own experiences and behaviour without getting emotionally caught up in them. This requires you to step back so that you can look at general patterns of emotional responses and learn to describe an emotion without being overwhelmed by it.

Imagine yourself trying to run a workshop on bereavement. If you have lost a loved one and still find it upsetting to think about this subject, then it's going to feel very personal and you might struggle to stay present in the teaching environment. However, by looking at the stages of grief (which generally apply to most of us) and how they play out in day-to-day life might in fact help you with your own situation. The part of our brain which we use to process rational thoughts like writing out a shopping list, or doing a maths problem, works separately from the part of your brain which processes emotions.

Training your brain to look at the process of grieving in a more academic and ultimately less personal way might enable you to observe your own experience with a better understanding of what is happening to you. The sadness of grief does not disappear, but the feeling of being disabled and overwhelmed by it diminishes. What's more, you're able to help others cope with their own loss in doing so.

And of course, there are other tangible harvests for people as well: securing a job or a flat, forging a new relationship, getting a dog, caring for an allotment, Louise putting on weight, Thomas losing weight, Anne getting stronger, Callum smiling when you crack a joke – or better still, Callum cracking a joke and making you smile – Miles arriving on time all week, and Mary getting her first certificate *ever*.

AFTER THE HARVEST

Work slows down as the gardening year draws to an end. You have some time to look at crop yields and decide what worked best and which practice needs to be revised. It is time to plan and prepare for the next season, order seeds for the spring, and collect and save seed from healthy plants. Some of these you can sow next year, some you can give away, or maybe swap for something you haven't tried yet that's been recommended by a fellow gardener.

It's also a time to reflect on what worked well for the people in the garden and what could be improved on, a time to take stock and look at all that has been achieved. Is Joe smiling more? Is Jenny getting better at time keeping? Has Tommy made some friends? Is Julie managing to keep on top of her alcohol addiction? These are the successes we routinely look for. In terms of what people achieve, the harvest sometimes feels astounding:

HARVESTING

Someone giving a presentation at a conference that moves people to tears and massively expands their understanding of mental illness and traumatic experience

The quiet volunteer who seldom speaks writing a beautiful article on the healing qualities of the garden for a magazine

People creating artwork of astonishing beauty

Simple acts of kindness from people who are struggling with their own demons but take the care to notice someone else's hardship

You can interpret all of this as seed dispersal – carrying the things learnt in the garden into new environments, exactly as it happens in nature.

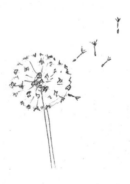

KEY POINTS

Harvesting

- A harvest can take anything from six weeks to six years. There are no rules; you have to be patient.

- People can achieve astounding results even while they are still unwell.

- We don't need to keep making the same mistakes: we can learn from them and do things differently.

CHAPTER 12

THE CIRCLE

The rhythm of the day. Driving to work at dawn in the early spring and watching the owls head home. Arriving at the garden when everything is quiet and catching the red flash of the fox disappearing over the wall; a family of stoats undulating across the drive, rabbits munching on the grass in front of the gates leading into the garden. Then, a cup of tea in hand, a walk round the garden before it wakes up and the bustle of the day begins. Experiencing the wonderful, unexpected smell of the viburnum on a cold winter's morning or the often-missed privet flowers (why do people always cut their hedges and miss out on that intoxicating scent?). Hearing the wonder of the frogs arriving back in the pond, as the noise of the ensuing debauchery reverberates all over the garden.

The excitement of planning the day. Shall we plant the peas out? Dig over the annual bed? Mow grass paths between the raised beds? There's the delight of sitting down together with a big sigh to have our picnic lunch after the effort of a morning's work. There's the satisfaction at the end of the day when we can see the progress that has been made – the tangible results of our labour. Going home nicely tired and looking forward to what we might do tomorrow. The garden always beckons us on to the next day, to the next task, to the next flower to break open, the next fruit ready to be picked.

THE RHYTHM OF THE SEASONS

There's the cycle of the wildlife. The birds mating, nesting and fledging. The heron flying over and the sparrow hawk being mobbed. The buzzards rising on the thermal currents above the garden. The gardeners hoping the rabbits don't find their way into the garden this year. Finding a mouse's nest in the compost heap. Hoping we don't get a wet spring and an invasion of slugs. The geese coming and going overhead, marking the seasons.

There's the cycle of the plants, too. Spring is a period of great activity, which starts in earnest in the greenhouse around the beginning of March, with annual vegetables and flowers being sown, trays of seedlings transplanted into single pots, and then later planted out into beds. The grass needs cutting, beds are dug over, perennials need staking, and vegetable beds need to be netted.

Moving into the summer months, the tasks involve weeding, cutting flowers, and harvesting the first crops of salads, peas, beans, raspberries and strawberries. There is a constant sparring with nature to keep pests and diseases at bay – constant vigilance is essential in an organic garden. But it's also a time when the pressure lifts and the garden is there for everyone to take pleasure in, with picnics, tea parties, and visitors during long warm days. It's a time for plant sales and relaxation, for letting the children play in this glorious green space. The presence of outside visitors is integral to the work going on in the garden.

I always start to feel sad towards the end of summer; I don't want to say goodbye to the warm days. But then comes the glorious spectacle of autumn, when the trees turn all the shades of yellow, through gold and purple to brown, and I am completely in awe of nature and this last fabulous firework display of the season. Autumn also brings the main harvest, such as potatoes, carrots, apples and pears, which all need to be stored against the winter months. A pleasant task is collecting seeds for the following year, before the birds carry them off to be dropped on fertile ground elsewhere. The birds are nature's original 'guerrilla gardeners', spreading seeds randomly, without waiting for permission, into many unlikely places.

People who are unfamiliar with gardens often assume that gardeners have nothing to do in the winter, but they couldn't be more wrong. In winter, the plants are dormant and don't mind being lifted and moved, so it's an ideal time to get busy and be creative.

All of the changes that need to be made, which you have observed throughout the year, can be done in those months. Because everything has stopped growing, you have the time to dig out and make new beds, reorganise beds or plants that aren't working, lay paths. It's a good chance to give the greenhouses a thorough clean out in order to get rid of any pests and diseases that might bring problems in the following season; a chance to paint the sheds and do lots of general tidying. Ironically, there is often no time in spring for a 'spring clean' in the garden.

In early winter, the tasks involve pruning fruit trees and hedges, lifting and dividing herbaceous plants, and moving them into their positions for the following year. Gardeners are always looking forward to what they can do next, how they can improve the garden, what they can try next year that's new and exciting. What new veg or flowers are on the scene? Perhaps the fennel, with its tall, bronze-coloured foliage, can be shifted into the back of the flowerbed to see if that looks better? It's the time to spend days foraging in the woods with wheelbarrows to collect the great bounty of fallen leaves – it's like walking on sunshine – and building enormous piles to make leaf mould. These piles can take three years to rot down completely, so it's a real investment in the future, and it's a great job on a bright winter's morning.

Bonfires are perfect for the coldest days, to clear up any detritus of the season that can't be composted. They're great fun and everyone loves them; baking potatoes in the embers and roasting marshmallows on sticks.

Come Christmas, there is the cutting of holly, ivy and fir to make wreaths that celebrate the season. This provides work for everyone. The 'rather be outdoors in any weather' types can cut and collect the materials. The 'happy to do anything but preferably not in the freezing cold' types will often spend time bunching in the shed just chatting or listening to the radio, enjoying the quiet rhythm of the work. The artistic types who enjoy fiddly work might make up the wreaths.

Around this time, you might see the skeleton trees in the snow. I always forget how lovely and somewhat hauntingly poignant they are. It's as if they're saying, "Come out for a walk, never mind the cold, we are only resting, we are still just as beautiful."

After Christmas and the New Year, we can get the catalogues and garden plans out and start planning for the spring.

And if during the year a disaster happens – a plague of green fly, an army of slugs, a drought – it is the very essence of life on this wee planet that life forms will find ways to grow again. Healing and growth are the natural drivers of plant, animal and human life, and if we pay attention to that in the right ways, creating the best conditions for health, then that is what will happen. There is always next season, where we get to do it all again.

If a therapeutic garden is open to the public and they are actively encouraged to visit, then the garden can aim to become a learning centre for the whole community, in the fields of organic horticulture and mental health. By drawing people into the garden with its beauty and intrigue, you can dispel the fear and stigma experienced by people with mental health problems, and for those who work in a mental health service. People come to enjoy the garden and stay to talk about their own life issues, particularly their own mental health or that of their loved ones.

One day, a delivery arrived in a big truck. Our volunteers did the unloading and checked things off as per usual, so it took a wee while. The driver seemed to be taken with the garden, so I showed him round and told him a bit about what we did. Then I made him a cup of tea. The truck was empty but he didn't seem to be in a hurry to leave so I went and sat beside him. He started to tell me that he was really worried about his wife. He told me she was very depressed after the death of her mother, who had been a great support to the family. He was worried that she wasn't managing to look after their young children properly. He had never really come across a serious mental health problem before and he felt completely out of his depth. He clearly loved his wife and children, but he had no idea how to help them. We talked for quite a while and I was able to give him reading material to take away with him. I encouraged him to take his wife to the doctor and get some help. He seemed more at ease when he left, but I never saw him again. I don't know the ending to this story, although I hope it was a happy one.

THE GARDEN CURE

The winter months can stretch on, and the weather can be wet and miserable with short days and long dark nights. For most of December and January, I can arrive each day in the dark and leave in the dark, so I am very grateful my job takes me outside during the day. Contrary to expectations, attendance is usually higher in the garden in winter as people need to escape cold, dark, often lonely flats, and seek the comfort of work, companionship and purpose. Just the joy of being outdoors together and being busy lifts our mood.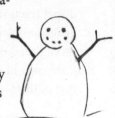

Every so often there will be a day of heavy snowfall which changes everything. It is like in Raymond Briggs' *The Snowman*[22] – a day out of time. You can raid the garden, build a bonfire, make soup and declare it officially a play day, sledging down the slope outside the garden, building snowmen and having snowball fights.

When the snow falls in a garden it creates a particular kind of beauty. It can give the people in it the opportunity to play again. This is hugely important in the life of someone experiencing long-term depression: a real day off.

As I said earlier, people are often frightened to have fun, in case those watching them think that they have only been pretending about how low they feel. Or else they have just forgotten how to enjoy themselves, so these times of fun and freedom can work wonders.

'In every walk with nature one receives far more than he seeks'

John Muir[23]

LIFE IS A VOYAGE, A JOURNEY

*"Push the boat out companeros, push the boat out
whatever the seas"*

Edwin Morgan[24]

The book, *The Tidal Model*,[25] which is referred to in earlier chapters, encourages you to picture life as a voyage. Once your boat building is complete, you set out to sail the oceans and have adventures.

Sometimes it is plain sailing, but at other times you hit the doldrums – a lovely metaphor, just like gardening – and you are stuck for a while. You might also be buffeted by a storm. If you are lucky, you will 'weather it' but if it is very severe you might be dashed onto the rocks.

At this point, you probably need help to get back to land. You will need to be rescued by someone who knows how to swim and, importantly, someone who knows how to manage a panicking, shipwrecked person who perhaps has never been taught how to swim. That rescuer has to have lifesaving skills, which can be learnt. He or she needs to be strong enough to take the weight of another person for a little while, and has to also understand that the person being rescued will be terrified and in total panic. The drowning person may well lash out at their rescuer by trying to grab hold of them, and may inadvertently pull them both under.

The rescuer has to be very firm at this point and take control: the person's panic will almost always subside once they feel held and supported and the rescuer can pull them to the shore. The ship itself can be brought back into dry dock and refitted. At that point, although it might show signs of repairs, it is ready to go back out to sea. As Phil Barker writes, 'a ship is safe in harbour but that is not what it was built for'. So off our intrepid traveller goes, out into the ocean for more adventures. Some will be good with smooth sailing and a fair wind, but inevitably they will hit a storm, be it a minor one they can cope with or a major one that will shipwreck them again for a while. Going back again into the dry dock for a refit is not a sign of failure, but of a life lived.

As I mentioned before, there is a lot of talk of 'revolving doors' in the mental health world. This refers to the occurrence of people who come back into services over and over again throughout their lives. In part, this can be caused by time-limited support, which is used as a kind of sticking plaster, a temporary repair, without allowing enough time to do a full refit. It is justifiably seen as a cause for concern.

People leaving the garden really appreciate the fact that they can come back if things get too difficult for them. In a situation where sufficient care was not taken in the building of the boat, we should surely rejoice in wonder that it can sail at all, and often so successfully, thanks to the courage and effort of the amazing sailor in charge? If it needs to come back for a few more refits than most, so be it.

The gardening year, like life's voyage, is a series of circles within circles. The garden moves from season to season, and each new year forgives the mistakes or mishaps of the previous one, giving us the chance to do it all again; to do it differently, to do it better. We can put the past seasons aside and learn from them without dwelling on them. We can look instead to the new season, with all its wonderful possibilities. We get to rewrite the story of the garden and our own lives within it.

THE CIRCLE

Part of rewriting the script can be your take on birthdays. Whatever we feel about them, they come around every year at the same time, just like snowdrops and leaf fall, and are a marker of our physical presence, our age, and our individual self. It should be a celebration of our unique part to play in the great dance of life, but many people hate their birthdays for different reasons. For some, they bring back memories of uncomfortable days with their families; for others, just being in the limelight in the smallest way can be difficult to deal with, as perhaps being noticed in the past might have led to being punished.

Some gardens like to have a routine of celebrating birthdays. They make sure that every single person on site, no matter what their role (paid staff can find it just as difficult to celebrate their birthdays), receives a birthday card, signed by everyone with kind wishes. They can sing 'Happy Birthday' (which people can opt out of if it feels too uncomfortable) and have a tea party at the end of the day, when everyone gets a fabulous homemade cake. For some people, it can be the first time in their life that they've had anything resembling a birthday party. For others, it has been a long time since.

In one community garden where I have worked for a few years now, it happened to be my birthday on our first Saturday open day (the plan was to have them once a month). Rather than miss it, I asked if I could just invite people and have my birthday celebration in the garden. Everyone loved the idea; someone made a big cake, others brought nibbles, and I received a lovely card signed by everyone. A big notice was put on the High Street inviting the public to join us which they did, and a good time was had by all. Since then, our monthly open day is dedicated to whoever has the closest birthday with cake, card, etc.

THE GARDEN CURE

I have seen many people moved to tears by the kind things people wrote in their cards, simple words of encouragement and friendship. I know most of us treasure our birthday cards from the garden. In the new script, birthdays are a day to celebrate the fact that people like and value you, and want to help you have a nice time, not a day to be fearful of or one that makes you feel bad about yourself.

The circles of my own life were not so different from anyone else's. There were good times, when everything sailed along nicely. There were times when I felt very low; when my youngest child very nearly died, when my mother passed away, when I suffered a serious back injury, when my elder child was involved in a hideous car accident – all of them ordinary human troubles. During these times, the garden and all its people and resources helped me get through it. There were joyful times when we could celebrate successes together, either on a public scale, like when we won awards, or on a very private, personal scale, like when someone who had never worked before was accepted onto a work training programme. This volunteer burst into the office with a huge look of surprise and delight on her face, and yelled "They want me!" And, of course, a tea party ensued.

Even in the dark depths of despair, something in the garden can catch your attention – the unexpected fragrance of a flower, the taste of a freshly picked raspberry, the colour of a rose in bloom, the winter wonderland of first snowfall, someone handing you a hot cup of soup on a cold snowy day. The beauty of working in nature constantly presents these opportunities for wonder and, just for a few minutes, lets in some light.

"Everybody needs beauty as well as bread, places to play in, places to pray in, where nature may heal and give strength to the body." John Muir

KEY POINTS
The Circle

- A garden beckons you into the future – the next season, the next cycle of growth.

- To make advances in mental health, you usually have to take some calculated risks.

- The joy of being outdoors and purposefully working together can help us through the dark days of winter.

- Healing and growth are the natural drivers of plants, animals and humans. Creating the best conditions for these drivers is more life-enhancing than focusing on treatment once the damage is done. Prevention is better than cure.

PART TWO

THE TOOL SHED

IN THE TOOLSHED

Gardeners love their tool sheds. If they don't have one, then they dream of it. The sight of all your tools looking clean, sharp and ready is a delight and an inspiration. I like to keep small tools like trowels, forks, secateurs, string and small knives in a wee bucket by the door so that I can grab them for a quick weed if I only have a few minutes to spare.

I like to have bigger tools like spades, forks and loppers hung safely on the wall, along with power tools: the mower, strimmer and hedge cutter. These tools are heavier and can be sharp, so they need to be treated with respect, both in the storing and the using. When I was a young adult and working in my first garden, I went into the large shared tool shed on the estate where I was living, which was very messy. It was cluttered and fairly dark and I walked into an Allen Scythe, which is a big cutting machine with rows of sharp blades on the front at ground level. I needed anti-tetanus, antibiotics and dressings for several weeks, but I learnt a valuable lesson about tool safety.

However, my ideal shed holds much more than just tools. It has a lovely pile of canes and nets and fleece ready to support and protect my crops. It also has a big Tupperware box filled with packets of seeds, with all their promise for the future, and piles of plant pots and seed trays just yearning to be filled. I keep a deep tray of sieved compost full and ready to go.

It has a shelf with a library of my favourite gardening books and seed catalogues, which I can dip into when I want inspiration, get stuck for ideas, or need a problem solved. It has a comfy chair and a wee stove; a kettle, mug and the tea-making things, and a biscuit tin for rainy days of reflection, planning, dreaming and relaxing. It is my oasis when I need some peace and quiet, and my magic carpet to visit plants from all around the world.

Oh, and it holds my radio to keep some contact with the outside world.

In this section, we will revisit some of the themes described in Part One, and here I would like to share some of the tools – the ideas, metaphors and techniques that have been useful to me and to the people I have worked with over the years.

They won't work for everybody on every occasion, so it is a bit of a 'suck it and see' approach.

The most important tool in a garden is yourself; spend time on keeping yourself well, focused and supported, i.e. in gardening terms, in a state of good repair. This will make your job so much easier. New people often start by asking lots of questions about illnesses that might affect other people, such as depression, anxiety or panic attacks. While it can be helpful to describe and know about these conditions, it doesn't usually help as much as you might think when you are actually working with people. Learning about the conditions and specific health problems of other people is important, but I found it was far more important to learn about myself. How I respond to stress, anger and distress, and knowing what keeps me well are of critical importance. I have to home in on how I deal with these things and hone my skills in managing my own behaviours and reactions. However, it can't be learnt in a day. It's a lifelong task; who we are, our life and work circumstances, our own physical and mental health, change constantly. We have to readjust continuously.

IN THE TOOLSHED

Like any good tool shed, this one is divided into broad compartments or areas so you can reach for what you need in any given situation. The three main areas here are:

HAND TOOLS: SIMPLE AND EASY TO USE
HAND FORKS, TROWELS, RAKES, SHEARS

These are relatively quick ideas anyone can use with just a little forethought and which are of real practical help. They are things you can try out if it feels right. You don't need lots of expert knowledge or outside help. Just give it a go, then discuss it with someone afterwards. Did the tool work? If so, how? Could it help in future?

POWER TOOLS: REQUIRING EXPERIENCE AND TRAINING
STRIMMERS, POWER MOWERS, HEDGE CUTTERS

These methods and ideas require a bit of study and expert help. Most of us don't start using a complex or specialist tool without assistance from someone familiar with that particular tool. Again, all have proved greatly beneficial and I've included references to useful resources should you wish to explore these further.

THE BOOKSHELF: THESE MIGHT ENCOURAGE YOU TO LOOK FOR A COURSE, AN EXPERIENCED PROFESSIONAL, OR FURTHER STUDY AND TRAINING

ARBORISTS, GARDEN DESIGNERS AND SPECIALISTS

This section covers the books (and articles and web-sites) we turn to for inspiration, those which have proved useful in a practical and theoretical sense. Pull them off the shelves when you need them, and look for an experienced practitioner, a class or course that will help you put them to actual use.

The number of tools I have included in each section could be smaller or greater. They all work for me personally and the people I have worked with. Just adapt and adopt as you see fit. Hopefully you'll find some inspiration as well as real pragmatic help in some of the handy hints and more in-depth ideas. I've found them useful along the way and now I hope you find your own ways to use them.

CHAPTER 13

HAND TOOLS

SIMPLE AND EASY TO USE

As every gardener knows, having good tools that are tailored to your size and ability, learning how to use them well, and keeping them in good repair are very important to the quality of his or her work. I am fairly small and have had a back injury, so working with a big spade doesn't suit me. I always choose a good border spade with a short shaft and a small, sharp blade; this way, I can dig much more safely than if I use a bigger, heavier spade. It might take me longer to dig over a bed, but I will get there without injury.

Learning to use any tool takes time, patience and lots of practice. Dougie MacLean, the Scottish songwriter, wrote a song for his young daughter when she asked him to teach her how to play a tune on the fiddle. The song is about when Dougie himself asked his father to teach him how to work the scythe, and it captures it beautifully.

O this is not a thing to learn inside a day
Stand closely by me and I'll try to show the way

You've got to hold it right
feel the distance to the ground
Move with a touch so light
until it's rhythm you have found
Then you'll know what I know[26]

(from 'Scythe Song', by Dougie MacLean)

THE GARDEN CURE

It always reminds me of trying to teach people to use a rake. It looks simple until you try it. You find yourself with big mounds of earth at one end of the plot and big hollows everywhere else. At that point you realise you need to learn 'the distance to the ground… with a touch so light'. The same goes for teaching the use of healthy-living tools: slowly and with a light touch.

Every gardener knows it pays dividends to spend a bit of time sharpening her tools, repairing any damage and replacing any broken shafts or handles.

It's not only a blunt tool that can do harm to a plant, but also the person using the tool in the wrong way. Making sure you know the correct way to use a tool is just as important to avoid damage. Sometimes it can be very hard to learn the right way if you have been practicing the wrong way for years. We all like to hold on to our habits even if they are damaging to us.

We must set aside old notions and embrace fresh ones, as we learn, we must daily unlearn something which it has cost us no small labour to acquire.
Homer, *Iliad*.[27]

The following are some simple to use tools that I found worked well for lots of people.

❋

164

1. ROUTINES FOR KEEPING WELL –
SLEEP, FOOD, HYGIENE, EXERCISE, COMPANY

Every gardener knows that routine is essential for helping everything stay healthy and well. I feed my plants on Mondays, making sure to clear away plant debris and clean and store tools at the end of each day, and so on. It is equally important to instil some healthy routines into our lives to help them stay in good shape. It saves us having to think everything through every day; we take time to plan a routine, then we follow it.

Recipes for good health are not very complicated but neither are they easy to put into practice. I have often met people coming into the garden feeling unwell both physically and mentally. Once I got to know them better, I might notice that they drank lots of coffee, skipped breakfast, and would have a can of coke, a packet of crisps and a bar of chocolate for lunch. Typically, they had very little energy or stamina, didn't socialise at all outside of the garden, and would stay at home playing video games for hours, watching movies or simply staring at the walls. None of this is conducive to physical or mental well-being.

However, habits are hard to change. Tackling one thing at a time can begin to make a difference, and once someone begins to feel even a very small difference, they are much more likely to engage with tackling more difficult life changes.

Often, people are genuinely oblivious to the negative effects of caffeine and sugar, and basic nutrition, so some explanations about that help too. People often say they have real trouble sleeping and consequently have trouble staying awake during the day. It turns out they are having about six to eight cups of coffee a day, washing it down with a large bottle of coke. It isn't the whole story of why they can't sleep, but it certainly doesn't help.

Sometimes in vegetable growing gardens, people use the produce to create a lunch club where you can pay a small amount and receive a bowl of homemade soup, fresh wholemeal bread, and a piece of fruit. Best of all, you do it together, so people slowly began to feel more comfortable about eating in public, which is often a difficulty. If it is just too tough, you can encourage people to serve the food instead – having a task really helps. Everyone has to take a turn in the kitchen, so people learn, or are reminded, how to make soup. You can also give people veg out of the garden to use at home. It is risky to try out new food on a tight budget. As discussed previously, if you are living on benefits then you are unlikely to have lots of money to spend on food. If you try something new and don't like it you don't have the money to buy anything else, so understandably people often stick to what they know.

Sleep hygiene can also be complicated on a tight budget. Accommodation can often be shared or very small, which can make sleeping areas cluttered and not restful. You can always try to encourage people to take small steps, just tackle one thing at a time. Many people have real problems about sleeping in a bed because of traumatic memories or fear of not being able to sleep. They might prefer to just stay on the sofa or on a chair in the living room in the hope of drifting off. If that is the case, it might be better to accept that is how it is, and to make that place as comfortable as possible. It's widely accepted that electronic screens stimulate the brain and prevent it from switching off at night, so perhaps encourage people to stop watching screens around nine or ten at night and see if that helps, especially if they have to be up at eight the next morning. Late at night, it might be better to listen to a radio programme or music instead. Some people find that having a light snack before going to bed – hot milk, not caffeine, helps them settle. If noise is a problem, try playing some background music or white noise to block it out. People sometimes don't feel safe enough to use earplugs or eye-masks. It is also suggested that sleeping with all your unpaid bills at the side of your bed might be a bad idea.

Gardening groups of any size need a system for managing domestic cleaning duties, as described earlier: the need to sweep and wash floors every day, wash dishes after every break, clean windows, and do the odd bit of paintwork every couple of months creates a level playing field. Everyone has to be involved, and people often shine in ways you might not have noticed otherwise. It also gives people that half hour of having to put their worries aside and do something physical. This is of great value when working with depression, and it establishes a routine of daily housekeeping.

2. WHAT TO DO TO RELAX WHEN YOU GO HOME – PLANNING FOR EMPTY TIME

If I am feeling anxious or worried about something, the worst time for me is when I have nothing to do, perhaps over a weekend. The empty time just leaves a space for my worries to multiply, and it helps if I make plans in advance to fill that time. Anxiety can make me forget how to look after myself properly, which leads to my mood getting even lower.

I usually feel purposeful and that I have achieved something at the end of a gardening session. This is a good frame of mind in which to plan the next phase of work, be it a session or a season. If I come into the garden without a plan, I can often spend ages walking around aimlessly, and I am less productive. By taking time to make a plan, I am less likely to feel overwhelmed by all that needs to be done, as I'll know when and how I will do it. Planning also ensures I bring everything with me that I might need to tackle specific jobs.

Sometimes, if I ask people what they have done the night before, a blank look will come over their faces and they will struggle to answer me. With a little more questioning it becomes clear that when they go home after a day in the garden they often do nothing at all. They can sit on the sofa and stare into space, perhaps for hours, until finally going to bed or, as often as not, just curling up to sleep where they are sitting. They just don't think or know how to look after themselves.

When this happens, it's productive to work together with the person to establish a routine for arriving home. This routine will help them relax, enable them to get through the evening, and prepare them for the next day. It's useful to write it down and pin it to a wall inside the front door. It might go a bit like this:

When I arrive home, I will:

Put some lights on

Hang up my coat

Put the heating on (assuming they can afford it)

Switch the kettle on for a hot drink

Put on the radio, music, or TV for some company

Start making some dinner (even if it's just beans on toast)

Decide how to spend the evening; preparation beforehand could involve having handy things like puzzle books, jigsaws, drawing materials, knitting, sewing, TV/radio programmes, library books, etc.

Phone a friend

Prepare clothes and make a packed lunch for the next day

Put a hot water bottle in my bed

And so on, personalising it to the person's wants and needs. Just having some rules so that you don't have to think things through and make decisions every night seems to be beneficial. Preparing for a weekend is equally important. Forty-eight hours by yourself, with a head full of worries and anxiety, can feel like a life sentence. But a bit of forethought can make all the difference. It might go a bit like this:

FRIDAY NIGHT: plan my meals for the week and make a shopping list

SATURDAY MORNING: go to the shops and buy what I need

Do laundry

SATURDAY AFTERNOON: go to the library/museum/free exhibition, or meet a friend

SATURDAY EVENING: meet a friend, go to the cinema, or one of the activities planned for weekday evenings

SUNDAY MORNING: prepare meals for the week ahead and freeze some portions

Sunday afternoon: go for a walk/meet a friend/work in the garden

SUNDAY EVENING: prepare clothes and a packed lunch for work the next day, relax with a book or TV, phone a friend

Even if you are on your own the whole weekend, it means you aren't looking at an empty expanse of time to get through, and you make it to the next week better prepared. Keeping busy helps with anxiety.

It is also worth encouraging and supporting someone to join group activities e.g. community adult education classes, yoga, walking groups, tai chi, reading groups, drama groups, a choir, a men's shed (community groups providing activities specifically for men), music sessions, or whatever suits the individual.

As has been shown throughout, people make friends more easily by doing things together. A chum on day one makes all the difference.

3. NOTICING THE ROUTINES THAT KEEP YOU WELL

I have little checklists for making sure everything is well in the garden. I check under the cabbage leaves to make sure there are no caterpillars lurking; I inspect the tomato plants for signs of greenfly; I stick my fingers into the soil to see if it's too wet or too dry; I keep a log of feeding the plants to make sure I do that regularly, and so on. In this way, I try to catch any problems in their infancy, before they become serious, as they are easier to correct.

It helps to make a chart of your own habits so that you can begin to recognise if your routines for staying well are in good shape or are slipping. Then you can catch it while you have the capacity to do something about it. Break it down into categories that are relevant for each individual. Here is an example of one such pattern. The idea is not to be judgemental – a problem for one person will not be an issue for another – but to notice the difference in behaviours.

4. PLAN FOR KEEPING WELL

INDICATORS	WELL	LESS WELL
Eating, Making meals	Planned meals, Fresh veg	Snacking: toast, chips, etc.
Sleeping	Seven or eight hours	Late nights, waking up at night, sleeping in (weekdays), less than six hours sleep
Seeing Friends	Planning meet-ups	Not bothering; staying home alone
Exercise	Daily walk, yoga class	Sitting on the sofa all day
Smoking	None, or five a day maximum	More than 10 a day
Drinking	A glass of wine or beer with dinner at the weekend	Three or more glasses a day
Personal hygiene	Daily shower and clean clothes	Not showering or doing laundry
Planning outings	Looking forward to doing things	Cancelling plans
Knitting, crafts, woodwork	Having a project on the go	Nothing on the go; watching more TV instead

The big flags for myself are not making proper meals because my energy drops right down. If this goes on too long, then everything else suffers. Not swimming regularly has a bad effect on my back and can lead to a serious episode of pain and incapacity. Because I am watching it, I am more likely to do something about it as soon as I notice. I also alert my partner so that he notices and prompts me.

4. TIME MANAGEMENT

If you rely on impulse and get lured into doing the first thing that catches your attention in the garden, you will be less effective. You might decide to weed a bed and get really involved in it and do a perfect job. But when you are finished and look around the garden, you realise that the rest of the beds are smothered in weeds and the plants you are trying to grow are suffering. With a little time taken to look around and plan, you might have decided to do an overall rough weed blitz to remove the worst offenders from the whole garden, before settling down to do a perfect job on any bed. Looking around also gives you the chance to think about the tools and equipment you might need. Planning how to use your time and energy efficiently yields much better results.

Learning to manage your time effectively is key to getting some control back into your life. If you can't get to where you want and need to go, then you can lose out, missing meet ups with friends, benefits agency appointments, which might result in loosing income, and even therapy appointments. Professional medical and psychiatric personnel are notorious for taking people off their lists if they don't show up for appointments, and to be fair, they can't work with someone who isn't there and their loss of time costs money. Likewise, the first things an employer wants to know about you are

punctuality and attendance. It's worth working hard on punctuality and timekeeping in the garden if you think you might
need a reference at some point or want to start regular employment. If someone can get on top of that, then it can open lots of
doors for them, not just in getting treatment, but socially and
in the world of employment.

Sometimes, people just don't seem to understand the
basics. For example, if we assume most people need eight
hours sleep each night, then you have to actually put aside
eight hours to be in bed. When someone is habitually late,
you might ask them to write a timetable of their week including all their activities over twenty-four hours each day. It is
then often clear that, while they understand that they are
expected to be on site by 9am ready to start, and while they
want to do that and are genuinely distressed when they miss
it because they have overslept, they are still out with friends
or up watching videos or playing Xbox until 1am. Of course,
there are usually very good and often complicated reasons
why people find it difficult to get to sleep, or indeed why they
might wake up during the night and can't get back to sleep;
reasons which lead them to avoid the issue as long as possible. These factors might need to be addressed if they do want
to get in on time.

For instance, if you have to start at 9am, you might need
to leave the house at 8.30am, and that means getting up at
7.30am to wash, have breakfast, and sort your lunchbox and
anything else for the day. Therefore, you need to be in bed by
at least 11.30pm, or better yet, 11pm. In order to get to sleep
by 11.30pm, you might have to be home or to stop watching
screens by around 10pm in order to have a shower, lay out your
clothes for the morning, and pack your bag. So, the decision to
be on time in the morning starts halfway through the evening

or maybe even at tea time the day before. Using a weekly time management plan, where you have to put in times for laundry, shopping, cooking, seeing friends and family, community activities and exercise can be immensely beneficial to some people.

The issues around getting out of the house on time may not be so simple or straightforward but one recurring theme for people who are socially anxious is worrying about what to wear, and many people spend ages trying to decide this every morning. It has nothing to do with vanity but is a deep-seated fear of not getting it right, looking odd or foolish, or standing out in some way.

It might help to try to encourage such people to spend the weekend deciding on a wardrobe for work. In the garden, we mostly wear old clothes that we don't mind getting dirty. Once they have decided on maybe three pairs of trousers and jumpers, and maybe five T-shirts, then these can be laid aside, clean, on Sunday for the week ahead. A trip to the nearest charity shop can be made if people are short of clothes, and dungarees are always a great choice to wear on top. It just needs some forethought and planning, and it means you no longer have to work it out each day.

It's the same with the packed lunches: plan them on Friday night, buy the ingredients on Saturday, and make them up the night before. It doesn't sound like rocket science, I know, but when we get really anxious, we often just need a bit of help to tap into the part of our brain that does organisation.

Anxiety on leaving the house is not so easy to manage for some. Many people can cope with the getting ready bit but then just can't get out of the door. I like to be in the garden a good hour before everyone else arrives so I can offer a phone-in routine in the morning (a friend could do this equally well). It might go a bit like this:

If Jenny is up and ready to leave but just can't get out of the house because she is too anxious, she can text me. I can then call her back (in case she doesn't have much money left on her phone) and chat on the phone for a bit: "It's a nice clear day, we thought you might like to plant the potatoes today or help put up the new fence." This will start a dialogue with her that makes her use her rational brain and think beyond the journey in. When I have got her talking, I might ask her just to open the door and sit for a minute and chat some more about work. When she seems a bit more relaxed, I can suggest she starts walking to the bus stop, all the while chatting about the day ahead. This can continue on the bus and all the way into the garden.

Soon, it might progress to just a call in the morning to help her out the door. She might send me a text from the bus stop, and I can call again for a wee chat while she is waiting. Then, if she is anxious on the bus – sometimes people have to get off the bus two or three times on even a fairly short journey – she can text again and I can chat. It doesn't usually take many days support for it to wind down to a single text just to reassure her we are there, or perhaps an occasional call if she has a panic attack and needs someone to talk to.

Another interesting discovery I've made is that often people don't use a diary.

Pete had very poor reading skills, not through lack of ability but through not having been able to attend school regularly during a sad and disruptive childhood. He had a very busy home life with four children and a partner who ran her own hairdressing business from home. He acted as his wife's secretary and accountant but was forever missing appointments himself and getting days wrong, and this upset him greatly. So, he worked with another volunteer to improve his reading skills. This went well and he became a very competent reader. However, he had never been shown how to use a calendar or appointment book, and so he tried to remember everything in his head. He thought everyone did that! Learning to use those tools was quite life changing for him and his children.

Time management often seems especially difficult for people with dyslexia and I was lucky enough to have the input of a specialist tutor who taught me how to use colour coding to make diaries and calendars easier to manage. She also taught me about **mind mapping,**[28] which proved to be an amazing tool that benefits everyone.

6. MAKING A START – LEARNING TO PUSH YOURSELF A LITTLE BIT MORE

When I moved into my house, I inherited a hideous concrete block double garage that took up a large amount of the garden and absolutely dominated it. The roof leaked and it wasn't even a useful storage space. I had two young children and a new full-time job and so, while I hated it, dealing with it went on hold for many years. I had also badly injured my back at the time and had very much lost confidence in my physical ability to tackle such a demanding job. The leaks got much worse and after many years we realised that, as the roof was asbestos and beginning to deteriorate, we would have to have it professionally dismantled and removed. That done, we were left with the concrete shell. By this point, I was at last building up the gumption to get rid of it, so I advertised it on lots of local web sites. Lo and behold, a friend wanted it, and swiftly took it apart and removed it. At last I was free to design the garden the way I wanted it, without this huge black cloud hanging over it. If only I had started the process ten years earlier.

When Jill first came to the garden, she had been ill with a debilitating disease. To start with, we waived the usual rules of that particular garden about attending three days a week and said she could come two short days a week instead. To start with, all she had to do was get there, then she could have a rest and go back home. She agreed to this and began to come to the garden. Slowly, as she made progress, she built up to three days, gradually staying for a little bit longer each week. It took her nearly twelve months to build up to three full days, and she often needed to rest for a bit each day, but eventually she regained her stamina and returned to better health. I have met several people who had a similar condition to Jill but they did not make the progress she did. So, I asked her what she thought had helped her.

She said she always went to the end of the road before she decided whether she was well enough to come to the garden or not. She felt if she got to the that corner, she would know whether she was genuinely too tired and unwell to come or just "couldn't be arsed". She said because she made herself get to the corner – which was the hardest part motivationally – before she decided, there were many more days that she made it to the garden. On multiple occasions, if she had made the decision when she woke up, she would just have stayed in bed.

When I hurt my back and had to spend years in recovery, a friend leant me a book which talked about "an aggressive approach to pain" and it made a big impression on me. Up until then everything I had read had said things like, don't push yourself too much, listen to your body and rest, be careful not to overdo it. (I appreciate this approach is not right for every condition, but at that time in my recovery it made me think about things differently.) I began to try not to give in to the pain all the time and started to at least plan to do more: concerts, days out, meetings with friends, etc. I didn't always make it or if I did get there I didn't often last through the whole event, but the intention was there and that began to make a difference. This 'get to the corner' mind-set often helped me to manage what I could do to get better. It prevented me from staying home each day and not making any plans.

7. NOTES TO FRIENDS: WHAT HAPPENS TO ME, WHY, AND HOW TO HELP

Companion planting: remember we talked about spending time with people who believe in you? Good friends want to help. You can make it easier for them by telling them a bit about your problems and what they can do to help. After I hurt my back, I learnt that the best way to keep it well was lots of vigorous exercise, and, of course, I needed to be working in a garden. This was an absolute essential for my well-being as well as being my job, no matter how incapable I was physically. For a while my dear friends and colleagues were so solicitous whenever I tried to do anything, as they were afraid I would hurt myself, that it felt like it was undermining my resolve to ever get better. I would often respond, I'm ashamed to say, with snapping at them to let me be. It got much better when I was able to explain to them that I had taken expert advice and was told that I needed to exercise my back regularly to build up the muscles. Just sitting watching would in fact make my condition much worse. I then promised to ask for help if I needed it, which I periodically did during a bad episode, but gradually my back did improve, and my friends got on board with the plan.

Some people have recurring problems, which can be disabling in their own right. This can be compounded by the effect these problems have on an individual's friends and by the way their friends sometimes react. With a little preparation, friends can do a lot to help. Usually, they are just frightened for you because they don't know what is happening or how to help.

Terry had frequent epilepsy seizures. All of a sudden, she would stop being responsive and seem to lose consciousness, and she would start shaking violently. It could last for several minutes and could look quite alarming, when she woke up she was often quite confused and disorientated for sometimes up to half an hour or more. Often, friends were wary of going out with her because they were afraid of the responsibility.

After some discussion, Terry prepared a letter to give to all of her friends so that they were better prepared and would understand what she wanted them to do and what would help her. It took away the fear of the unknown and gave them the confidence to offer the right support when needed. It might go a bit like this.

Dear friend, here are some things I would like you to know:

What happens to me sometimes: I have seizures which happen suddenly. They look really serious, as if I am having a heart attack, or a stroke, but I am unlikely to be medically ill.

What it looks like: *I will pass out and I might start shaking violently and be unable to speak or respond, although I might be able to hear you some of the time especially as I come round. Afterwards I might not remember what happened and be a bit confused for a while.*

What I need you to do: *Make sure I am in a safe place. Keep talking to me quietly and reassure me that I am safe. Loosen any tight clothing if it's safe to do so. Put something soft under my head to stop me banging it. Don't let people crowd round me. Stay with me and keep me calm for at least 30 minutes after the symptoms have subsided. Talk to me about it another time, when I am calmer. Keep me warm and out of danger, and please keep others away. I will probably want to go home but make sure I am fully recovered before you leave me.*

What I don't want you to do: *Don't panic yourself. It can look quite alarming. Don't immediately call an ambulance, unless I don't come round within 5 minutes, or I seem to have hurt myself falling. Don't try to force anything into my mouth. Don't try and get me to problem solve when I come round because my brain will not be working well enough to do that. Don't give me caffeine but offer calming herbal teas or water.*

This letter worked for this individual, though it should not be used as a general letter for anyone with epilepsy. Similar adapted notes might work for someone with asthma or panic attacks or fugue attacks (during which the person will appear to be conscious but is actually absent; they might seem unresponsive and spaced out with glazed eyes, and they might not recognise where they are). If friends know and understand what is happening, they are much more likely to be helpful and supportive and less afraid of the situation.

8. 'AND' NOT 'BUT' – ENCOURAGING PEOPLE TO AIM HIGHER

Most plants don't do well in the shade. Let the light shine on them and watch them blossom.

I was once sent to a three-day training course for managers. It was very high powered and focussed a lot on image and making an impression. I only remember two things the trainer said. The first was that the speaker should be the smartest-dressed in the room. Well that was never going to fly. However, the second was very powerful:

'And' not 'but'. The example the trainer gave was a scenario where she asked her administrative worker to prepare her a full report on X for Friday afternoon. It didn't land on her desk until the Monday morning. She had the choice of two responses to her admin worker after reading the report.

a. Thank you for the report on X. It was very thorough and well written, but it was late.

b. Thank you for the report on X. It was very thorough and well written, and it would be even better if next time it was completed on time.

Our brain processes the words 'and' and 'but' quite differently. If she had said the first sentence, then all the worker would hear is "it was late". By using the second sentence, the worker manages to process the praise as well, and is motivated to do better next time.

I loved it. It was so simple. I try to use it whenever I need to impart anything of a critical nature. Inspiration to do better works much better than a telling off for getting it wrong.

9. TALKING ABOUT TRAUMA

I was recently working in a very old garden trying to rejuve-
nate aged and battle-scarred apple trees. One in particular
was so overgrown, that it clearly hadn't been pruned in many
years. It had huge wounds in the base, had lost limbs, and
there was a big hollow in the trunk. I thought it was time for
it to go and was set to cut it down. For some reason I decided
to wait and see how it performed over the year, so gave it a
good prune and a feed and waited. Lo and behold, come the
summer and against all the odds, it produced a great crop
of fruit. It's amazing what trees and people can survive with
good support.

Sometimes people who have been abused or neglected as
children are taught since very early on that they are responsible
for the bad things that happen to them. They grow to believe
that if they ever tell anyone or if anyone finds out, then there
will be severe consequences: the shock might kill their mother,
no one will believe them, or they will be taken away and put
in a home.

Of course, a young child has no option but to believe these
lies as they are coming out of the mouth of an adult – often
one the rest of the world values and respects – and so they do
their best to keep it all secret. The fear of what might happen if
anyone finds out feels impossible to live with. This has drastic
effects on their behaviour and beliefs as it denies them access
to other adults who might be able to help and support them.
Sometimes it can take half a lifetime for someone to feel confident enough to discuss childhood traumas.

When they do, it can feel as if they have stepped into a
different universe. Suddenly, from feeling in control of that
information with everything being locked up inside them, they
are plunged into a world where someone else knows and has

that control. I remember one man describing it as feeling like a huge, heavy cloud had appeared and was going to smother him. It took three days and a lot of persuading to urge him to come back to the garden after he had told me what had happened to him.

The moment of disclosure can be a confusing and bewildering time for an individual. They are in a state of shock and often don't understand why it is that they feel so vulnerable. Why don't they feel better for sharing the load? Most of us believe that talking about things helps, so it's a shock when it does not seem to immediately. It's an important moment to recognise the conditioned thinking that comes with abuse – to recognise the perceived need for secrecy and feelings of guilt – and to challenge it. All of this has to happen at a time when someone who has been brave enough to explain past traumas still does not know or understand the rules the rest of the world lives by. I would use the analogy of flat earth thinkers described previously to help people understand their own feelings and responses to being in a world where all the rules have suddenly changed.

10. MISERABLE AND USEFUL – WORKING WITH LOW MOOD

Often in the garden, someone will arrive clearly upset. It might be a bereavement, a worrying health diagnosis, a child deciding to emigrate, a bill that can't be paid or struggling with an ongoing low mood and depression. It helps when people can come and share these things with someone who will listen sympathetically. But what helps more is when, having discussed the problem, that person can busy themselves doing something useful in a beautiful place with supportive friends.

Coping with depression is a truly miserable experience and can be crippling. People also worry, as I've said earlier, that if they appear to be able to do practical things, then others might not believe how bad they actually feel. So sometimes they will demonstrate how awful they feel through their behaviour. Sadly, this becomes a self-fulfilling prophecy. If you can persuade that person that you understand how bad they're feeling and that it might actually help if they do something useful – and you understand that they will still feel just as miserable and are not lying or exaggerating their condition – then they might begin to feel better about themselves..

If I can explain this notion that the alternative to being 'miserable and useful' is 'miserable and useless' most people get it and start to fight the depression by becoming more active, even while having to overcome the belief it won't help them feel better. They see that, even if you still feel miserable, it's better to be useful rather than useless. Then, of course, it does actually work, because if you have done something useful today, however small, you feel just that wee bit better about yourself, and eventually your confidence begins to grow. You may still feel depressed and anxious but feeling that you can contribute and therefore have a useful place goes a long way to starting the healing process. A garden full of meaningful work-focussed activity makes that possible.

11. LOOKING FOR THE 'THIRD OPTION' – A MAGICAL WAY OUT OF YOUR PROBLEMS

"Back to my garage: I just wanted it to go away and moaned about it – for over ten years. It wasn't until I took the only effective course of action that I got the result I wanted."

Terry Waite[29] wrote that when he was taken captive, he spent a long time raging about his situation (which was a truly horrendous hostage situation). Then he made a breakthrough in his thinking. He realised that raging about what was and longing for it to be different didn't actually change anything. It was wearing him out in a dangerous way. All of his energy was spent on hating where he was and what was happening to him, and wishing it were different. Then he realised he was looking for something that was not there, and if he continued this way he was unlikely to survive. He told himself he had three options:

- Change your situation

- Change how you respond to your situation

- Look for something else that would somehow resolve the situation

He realised that he had been fervently depending on the third option. He was powerless to change his situation as he was a prisoner under armed guard and had explored all escape options. 'Something else', the one he was waiting for, just didn't exist or if it did, he had no power over it. However, he could do something about the way he responded to his situation. He could meditate, practice yoga and change his state of mind. He writes of trying to remember in detail memories of whole days in his mind to pass the time. He had to do whatever would help him stay calm and survive this ordeal he found himself in. He could and did change the way he responded to his situation, and miraculously saved his sanity.

It reminded me of Mairi, who would arrive upset most days because she had noisy upstairs neighbours. She had suffered their noise for several years and was anxious and upset by their behaviour. She was so stuck in her anxiety that even when they weren't throwing a noisy party she would stay awake all night listening just in case they did. She was set on waiting for the third option to get her out of this situation. She wouldn't consider trying to change the situation by applying for a housing transfer, which would have been possible, or approaching the tenant reconciliation scheme, or by finding ways of cancelling out the noise, like earplugs or white noise. She just kept on wanting something to happen to make it stop.

It took a long time working with Mairi to encourage her to look at options where she had some control. I think we all get stuck trying to find third options from time to time. When I hurt my back, I spent ages hoping to find someone who would make it better for me. Of course, the problem with the third option is that we are probably looking for something that is simply given to us – the magic pill or the brilliant miracle-worker or therapist. Whereas we might certainly benefit from some form of medication and from help from an appropriate therapist, the process still requires us to do lots of difficult work for ourselves.

After my back had begun to heal and I had returned to work and was managing my life a bit better, I used to get phone calls from people – friends of friends – who had been given my number, hoping I could help. They would say: "I've got a really sore back and so and so said you had too, but that it got better. What was it that helped?" I would say: "I did back exercises every hour and swam three times a week." They would respond: "But I have a really sore back and I don't know what to do", and so on. They were as stuck as I had been, and it took me a long while to realise it. You have to be ready to hear the message about taking responsibility for yourself, because it's not what you want to hear, and it can be difficult and painful.

12. COMFORT BOX – TIPS FOR GETTING THROUGH LONELY HOURS

I suspect that for all of us who work in gardens, there are days when you just don't have the energy. That's when you are glad you took the time to put in a bit of a sheltered space with some nice planting, a table and chairs, maybe a wee corner of the greenhouse where you also store some gardening books. Allow time for a rest.

Some people find it helpful to put together a comfort box, for times when they feel especially low or for the moment they wake up during the night and need something to calm themselves. What goes in it is very individual, but things which might appeal to the senses, like a nice stone or a smooth piece of wood from a place visited and enjoyed, can be useful. You can hold such an object in your hand, or you could have a small piece of silk that feels soft, or a scarf that feels warm. Favourite sweets, something scented like lavender or cinnamon, photographs of good friends and happy times, CDs, uplifting poetry or short stories, a crossword or puzzle book, funny cards that remind you of friends, a wooden puzzle or jigsaw, a non-news related magazine on a favourite hobby, and so on. Any of these can provide comfort and distraction from current sadness, and are ready at hand when you are not able to think beyond the present.

13. POSTCARD WALL – TIPS FOR LIFTING LOW MOOD AND LONELINESS

In my garden, I especially treasure things given to me as gifts from friends and family: the rose arch sent for my birthday from my daughter in Australia, the planters and tulips from my other daughter in California, and all the plants which I have swapped with friends. They are great additions to my garden but have extra value because of the love they symbolise. When I am missing my daughters, I just need to take a walk round my garden and it feels as if they are close by.

Here is a simple idea to remind people that they are not alone, that they do have friends and people who care about them. Ask people to keep any cards they are sent from friends and family for birthdays, holidays, etc. and put them up on a wall where they are regularly seen. In the garden, we always give people a birthday card, which everyone signs with messages of friendship and good wishes. People find that on a bleak night it is good to have these on a wall in their bedroom, so they're able to get back in touch with the feeling of being valued. I have a wall covered in funny cards people send me in my bathroom, which never fails to cheer me up. It's an added delight when people new to our house ask to use the bathroom, then five minutes later you can hear them chortling away to themselves.

14. RELAXATION TECHNIQUES

Gardens are great places to relax - not necessarily by doing nothing. It's often the simple repetitive weeding of a path or bed that I find most relaxing.

Relaxation techniques are really useful for people who can learn them and use them, but caution is needed when working with trauma. People with severe trauma in their history have often been in situations where they were not safe, where bad things happened to them, where their living situation was inherently dangerous. Sometimes this lasts for many years. It is no surprise, therefore, that they often develop PTSD (post-traumatic stress disorder) and become 'hyper-vigilant'. Like a war combatant, they have lived in dangerous situations and have learnt, often at their cost, that it pays to be very aware of everything around you. They've learnt not to let their guard down for a minute. So if they go into a relaxation class, which, being a largish group, will often feel very threatening anyway, and the tutor says something like: "Try to remember a time when you felt totally safe and relaxed...", "I would like you to close your eyes...", and "I would like you to lie on the floor...", they are unwittingly describing postures of helplessness and vulnerability. For some individuals, they have no memories of a safe place.

A good teacher will strive to understand a person's background and will find ways of working around these obstacles, but it can require a fairly specialist level of expertise. It's worth trying to meet up with the teacher before you attend the class, to explain how you might feel or react.

Finding an absorbing physical activity with an engaging mental component such as pruning fruit trees and bushes, can distract such an individual from their constant state of worry and fearfulness, and can sometimes work well as a relaxation tool. Partly, this is because they have to keep moving. The other aspect is that they have to look at what they're doing instead of constantly scanning for danger.

15. MAKING YOUR MARK – HOW ART AND CREATIVITY CAN MAKE A DIFFERENCE

Nowadays, it is widely accepted that there are no such things as weeds – just plants growing where we humans don't want them to. Everything in nature deserves its place. How many times have you seen rogue poppies springing up where you didn't sow them? I love them all the more for their defiance in growing where they're not supposed to be. They make their mark with beauty and determination, and I always leave them be.

In the various gardens I have worked in, I have been very fortunate to have met several experienced art teachers among the volunteers, who generously offered their skills. They gave art lessons, ran art workshops, organised exhibitions, supervised the creation of group murals and sculptures, and generally brightened up our lives.

Freddie ran an art group to make some very large outdoor murals. The individuals involved were so excited with what they had achieved. These were people who had never rated themselves highly or been recognised for any outstanding skill or talent, and here they were, creating something that was going on public display and was highly praised by everyone who saw it. The art tutor talked about letting people 'make their mark'.

It made me think about my life as a gardener. Is it the same need to make a mark that fuels enthusiasm for gardening and other creative work? You put something you have created on public display and wait for the reactions.

I was working recently in a public community garden with a small group of volunteers. I decided we needed to build a small retaining wall to stop soil eroding down the slope of the main flowerbed. We had just been donated lots of willow, so I showed the volunteers how to build a willow fence. It was only about four yards long and about a foot high, but they were so happy to have learnt to construct something new that was also pleasing to the eye. It was going to be there as a feature for a couple of years and viewed by many visitors. Their pleasure in this was an unexpected delight.

You work away and at the end you have created something and it's there for all to see.

16. THE MIRACLE QUESTION – HELPING PEOPLE BECOME UNSTUCK

Often, there is quite a gap between what I want a garden to look like and what it is now. It's easy to be daunted by what seems like an impossible amount of work. Breaking it down to one area, bed, task or tree at a time makes it possible for me to complete the job at hand and gives me the confidence to take on the next task.

Solution-focused therapy[30] is a way of working with people that focuses on what the person wants to achieve, rather than exploring their past and how it has influenced them. In order to deliver this kind of therapy, the practitioner would normally undergo a fairly lengthy training process.

However, a really simple and powerful notion from it is what is often called the 'Miracle Question'.[31] This encourages the individual to try to envisage what their life might look like if their current problems were resolved. "Imagine that you go home tonight as usual, do what you normally do and then go to bed and fall asleep. While you are sleeping, a miracle happens, and all your current problems are resolved. When you wake up you don't know about the miracle but are aware that things are different. It might be some small things or a whole lot of things. Can you describe the changes you see?" People might at first reply that they don't know, so it takes a bit of time to explore this idea. Then they might say something like: "When I woke up, I wouldn't feel scared." The counsellor might then spend sessions working out how this can be achieved.

> I worked with one group of volunteers to learn about SFT (Solution Focused Therapy), and Larry in particular sticks in my memory. He got very excited by the miracle question and started filling a notebook with what his life would look like if he felt better. It included lots of detail on where he would live, the colours of paint on the walls, and so on. When he showed me the list of what would be different, I noticed one of the things on his list was that he would have a dog. I asked him if there was something preventing him from having one now. He looked at me in silence for a long moment and started to smile then said: "No there isn't!" The following week he went and adopted a rescue dog. It was great to see just that little bit of control come back into his life and it was the first of many things that improved for him.

17. PANIC ATTACKS

Plants don't exactly have panic attacks in the same way that humans do, but they can suffer from many other kinds of attacks and can go into shock. Aphids, caterpillars, slugs, weevils, extreme heat or cold, under or over watering can all attack a plant's system. Once you understand the cause and effect of the attack it's much easier to get on top of it.

Panic attacks are much more common than most people imagine. It is really useful to do some reading on what is actually happening and the best way to help. People often look as if they might be having a heart attack. Typically, the person becomes very agitated and not able to communicate well. Symptoms might include: racing heart; feeling weak or dizzy; tingling or numbness in the hands and fingers; fear of dying; feeling sweaty or chilled; chest pains, shallow breathing, struggling to breathe; feeling out of control and feeling sick. It can truly feel quite terrifying, as if you're in a plane and have just been told the engines have caught fire and that you need to assume the crash position.

The most important thing to do to support someone having a panic attack is to stay calm yourself, learn the protocols and gain an understanding of the physiological causes of panic attacks. In a calm moment you can help people learn about these causes, which often relate to the flight, fight or freeze response. They can be reassured that it will not physically harm them and that it can be controlled with practice.

Janet suffered from severe panic attacks. When the feelings of panic and 'overwhelm' felt very severe, she thought she was having a heart attack. She couldn't breathe, and felt she was going to pass out or even die. The urge to run away from the situation at hand was strong. However, this would give a clear message to the brain that the situation you're in is truly dangerous and reinforce the fear, even if you are only standing in a queue at the supermarket.

For Janet, feeling trapped in a queue in a busy shop was a very common cause of panic attacks. When the attack was over, she could see that she was in no immediate physical danger in the store. The real fear she was experiencing was to do with her emotional state. She would break down and start to behave strangely, maybe trembling and crying, in her desire to be out of the shop and at home. People would then crowd round her, trying to help but making her feel exposed, overwhelmed and much worse. She was amazed that in this awful condition we would ask her to stay where she was, maybe just to move to a quieter part of the store with her back against a wall (so that no one could come up behind her). That way, she could give us a call so that we could calm her down by going through the panic attack protocol.

It always seems to help those suffering from panic attacks to speak to someone who is familiar with managing them. If you're acting as the support, you can talk the individual through the exercises to help reduce panic, like standing with their back against a wall. You can help them to calm their breathing, which is probably fast and shallow; sometimes breathing into their hands or a paper bag can help. Remind them that they have survived panic attacks before and will do so again. When they begin to calm down, you can try to engage their rational thinking brain by asking questions about their surroundings – "What colour is the car parked nearest to you?" "Is there a bus coming towards you, what number is it?" and so on, until you are sure they are back in control. Gradually people can learn to apply the technique by themselves, but it does require that first step of riding out terrible fear. Once that fear has been con- quered, the next panic attack seldom has quite the same grip. Once people understand the mechanism of panic attacks, they can often get on top of them fairly quickly. They will probably still experience the fear and anxiety but will be able to manage the physical symptoms better.

18. MAKING A POSITIVE CONNECTION

The best way to help someone understand a plant's needs is to give them one to take home and put in their own garden. They make a connection with it and come to appreciate its strengths and beauty. They learn which aspects suit it best; how much water it needs, how much feeding, how it tastes when it's picked fresh, and how resilient it can be when faced with appalling weather conditions. Without that connection and understanding, it is difficult to work through vulnerabilities and to understand strengths.

When people first come to a therapeutic environment, they usually resort to the medical model that they're used to and want to tell you about their symptoms and problems. While this is understandable, and while it will prove necessary at some point in helping them recover, it is really important to try and discover a positive connection.

I spent a long time talking with a new woman, Jenny, who explained at length the depth of her distress. It was based on horrendous childhood trauma. She said she longed to depart this life which was so hard for her. She was clear that she would only stay until her daughter was old enough to finish university and look after herself.

We talked for a while as I tried to gently see if there was anything positive in her life to build on. She was on the point of walking out the door when she suddenly said she was worried about her birds and would need to find some-one to take care of them.

I felt a huge sigh of relief, as I now knew how to begin to engage with Jenny. We talked about her birds and how she had lots of tame wild birds which came to her garden feeders, and she suddenly showed much more life and enthusiasm. I told her we had never had much success with feeding the wild birds (which was true) and asked if she might be prepared to advise us and set up a feeding station for us if I gave her a bit of a budget. And so, it began; she attended the garden with her own area of expertise and responsibility. It was a small step in her road to recovery but a very positive one.

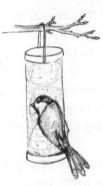

CHAPTER 14

POWER TOOLS

THESE NEED SOME EXPERIENCE, STUDY AND TRAINING

These ideas and frameworks are drawn from books and well-established practices. As with a power tool, you need to study the instructions carefully and spend some time learning how to use them. They are tools shaped by psychological theories, research, and explorations, or just plain experience of what works well. They are best used with a bit more background than the practical quick fixes; the bibliography and references which follow may be of help here. But these tools are also an aid to mental health and are available to anyone, with the proviso they put in some time to learn about them.

I. THE HUMAN GIVENS[32] (JOE GRIFFIN AND IVAN TYRELL) – A SOLUTION-FOCUSED FRAMEWORK FOR WORKING WITH PEOPLE

Every garden works better with a plan and a framework. Understanding where the light falls and the direction of the winds helps to discover the sheltered areas and the best spots for plants. What is important to you? What does the garden need to do? What do you want to grow – fruit, veg, trees or flowers? A structured assessment of the growing space helps to plan for growth more successfully.

There are many ways of working with mental health problems. Some methods focus on helping people to understand their past, the origins of their difficulties, and how you might learn to manage them better and reach some kind of peace. Other methods such as solution-focused therapies don't put so much emphasis on the past but rather on where the person is now and what they might have to do to achieve their desired goals in life, such as feeling less anxious, getting better at meeting people and forming relationships, or securing employment

The Human Givens approach falls into the latter category. It starts with the premise that all humans have the same basic emotional needs in order to thrive (assuming they have the basic human needs, such as a roof over their head, food and water, and physical safety).

When something is a 'Given' it means that most people would not dispute its truth. So, the Human Givens is a list of emotional needs we all have in order to flourish. Most of us can manage without some of them for a short while, but long term we would become emotionally unwell and exhausted without them.

Helping people meet these needs is a good basis for working out the principles of working practice. I found this a very positive way to work both in my own life and with other people. I don't have to know anything about someone's past, I just need to work with them to observe how they are feeling in the present. People can use the following list to assess for themselves how they are feeling about each area of their lives, by giving each a score out of ten, one being very poor and ten being very good. They will then know which area it will be useful to focus on. They are as follows, and with each is a description of how you can work with it.

FEELING SAFE AND SECURE ON A DAILY BASIS

There is seldom a lot you can do for people's home lives except try to help them become more confident and make wise choices when tricky decisions arise. But within a garden there is a lot you can do. (See above chapter on creating a safe place).

HAVING A SENSE OF COMPETENCE AND ACHIEVEMENT – FEELINGS OF SELF-WORTH

Being part of a beautiful garden can do a lot to promote a sense of achievement. Volunteers can take a real sense of pride in doing their part in building it and showing visitors round. Despite all that might have happened to them, they are able to give something back to the community. Many people have accompanied me to conferences and training days to tell their stories, as well as acting as tour guides when we have visitors to the garden, and chatting to passers-by, who happen to wander in.

HAVING A SENSE OF CONTROL AND INFLUENCE OVER EVENTS IN YOUR LIFE

Many people's lives were out of their control when they were growing up, causing them great distress. Sometimes volunteers are living on social security benefits, which means they have little control over their budget, which in turn affects their housing situation, their social life, diet, ability to buy new clothes, heat their home, and go on holiday. But there are other areas of life over which they might have more control. Getting a paid job is often what people present as their most urgent concern. While accepting this as a genuine goal, you can try and break it down into manageable steps e.g. punctuality, regular attendance and neat appearance, as many workplaces have a dress code of some kind and most like their staff to be clean and tidy. You can offer to provide a reference once these things are achieved. Small steps of claiming back control are useful before tackling big ones like problematic family relationships or controlling anger and fear.

FEELING CONNECTED TO THE WIDER COMMUNITY – HAVING A SENSE OF BELONGING

People do, surprisingly quickly, develop a sense of belonging. Whether the garden is part of a big mental health charity, who might refer to it as a training garden, or a small garden run solely by a handful of volunteers, the people working there will talk about it being a community, and nowadays there are many flourishing gardening communities in this country. There is something about working alongside each other in all weathers and having to overcome physical and technical problems (thus stretching each person's abilities) that seems to bind people very quickly. People will arrive in the most appalling weather when there is no likelihood of doing any gardening. One can only assume that they want to be together doing something useful, if possible, rather than on their own at home.

GIVING AND RECEIVING ATTENTION

This is a very interesting one and it's to do with different kinds of relationships. Some people have as many as eight people working for them from the social or psychiatric services. The topic is always the 'patients' themselves and what is going on for them: it's not a two-way relationship. The professionals are there to listen to what is happening to their 'patients': how they are feeling and how their lives are going. It is deemed very unprofessional for any of these practitioners to introduce their own well-being and home situation into the discussion. So, while individuals supported by mental health services are used to receiving lots of attention, they do not usually have the opportunity to give someone *their* attention.

Paid staff in a therapeutic garden must hold professional boundaries, but it is fundamentally a different situation. It is a *working* relationship as well as a therapeutic one. When you are working hard physically with people all day, you have to be able to depend on each other. If you are moving a heavy tree together, you have to be able to trust and rely on your colleague, or it becomes dangerous. It's difficult to hide what state you are in. There are no one-hour appointments and no breaks. People can see if you are not doing well. You might have a headache, a period, be worried about a child, have just received a big bill you can't pay, or be suffering from a sleepless night. While it may not be appropriate to go into details of why you are a bit under par, it would be hard, wrong, and probably impossible, to just pretend everything is fine for seven hours at a stretch. It actually does no harm at all to let people know that you are not made of resin or some impenetrable material, and that you too have bad days, and it makes the physical working practice safer. If a volunteer is offering to bring you a cup of tea, then thank them graciously and make sure they know your mood is in no way his fault, and that you appreciate his concern.

One of the questions I usually asked people who came to our visitors' days – if they are in one of the 'caring professions' – is what motivates them to do the job they do. They almost always say something along the lines of: "It makes me feel good about myself to be able to help other people". Letting volunteers have this opportunity to show some empathy and understanding, not just for each other but also, on occasion, for staff members, is surely a good thing. That is with the proviso that you give them information about yourself so that they understand it's not their fault if you are a bit withdrawn. They don't need any details and you must be clear in your own mind that if you feel it's appropriate to tell someone you're not feeling very well, you are doing so to let them know that your low mood has not been caused by them; it should not be about your own need to unload. When I returned to work after my back accident, the volunteers seemed to take it in turns to meet me from my car and carry my bags in for me. I didn't ask them to and I didn't discuss my back with them. They just did the kind, compassionate thing and I was suitably grateful because it helped.

HAVING TIME FOR PRIVACY AND REFLECTION

People who have grown up with no respect for their privacy can find this difficult to manage in a healthy way as an adult. One person may shut herself off in her flat or room, seldom venturing out, or only if she can be sure she won't meet too many people. She is the one likely to shop for groceries at 10 o'clock at night. For someone else, it might be the other way around; they're unable to keep people at arm's length. They find their privacy is constantly being invaded because they don't have the confidence to say no, or because they dread being alone.

Volunteers have to share space in the garden, so interpersonal boundaries need to be clear and respected. Sometimes jobs will allow people to work alone but most often they will demand at least some interaction with others. This can be a difficult learning situation for many, but with a large garden and lots of room, it is much easier to accommodate an individual's need for space than it would be in most workplaces. Knowing that a job has to be done and can only get done with other people's help, seems to make it easier for people once they grasp and embrace the purpose of the garden. It can help to establish a quiet area. A place, maybe a shed or a covered bower, where people can go when they feel overwhelmed or just need to be alone for a while. This can be a highly valued space for some people.

FEEL AN EMOTIONAL CONNECTION TO OTHERS

Feeling that somebody cares about you, notices when you are absent, is pleased to see you, even when you are having a bad day, and wants to celebrate your successes, however small, is very reassuring.

This can be a slow build when someone feels very negatively about themselves or has felt for many years that nobody cares about them at all. Sometimes you might have to teach, or remind, people what being cared about looks like. You might establish a routine of phoning people if they don't turn up and haven't phoned to tell you they aren't coming. You know people might feel hacked off with you pestering them when they are feeling low. There is always the danger that they might think you are having a go at them or are annoyed with them for failing to turn up. They may even think you are trying to rub it in that they have failed again. Balanced against what they might feel if you don't phone – "They didn't even notice I wasn't there; no one cares whether I am there or not" – it seems worth the risk. Occasionally, the call has proved to be literally lifesaving.

A SENSE OF STATUS – A VALUED ROLE IN SOCIETY

We are social beings and we care about how other people see us. People who are unemployed and have a mental health problem often perceive their own social status as being very low. This was why it is so important that a community garden, especially if it is a therapeutic one for people with mental health problems, shines as a vibrant place, recognised by the public, and valued by visitors and judging bodies in the horticultural as well as the mental health worlds. It should apply for lots of competitions, not because it needs the applause, but so that volunteers can feel pride in their connection to the garden and their role in its success.

Some of the people I have found most confusing to support were those who had worked in caring professions: doctors, social workers, psychiatrists, therapists. This was not because they were difficult people but because of the role reversal they were experiencing. Every day it felt as if they were having their noses rubbed in their loss of status. They used to be the people who did my kind of job and now they were on the receiving end, thrown into a world (of horticulture) they sometimes knew little about. Because of that, these individuals sometimes felt helpless and de-skilled.

When I first learnt about the Human Givens, I was working with a man called Ian, who had been an occupational therapist. He found it very difficult to work with our system. I had tried everything I knew to engage with him. He would always come in late so he missed the morning briefing sessions for the day's jobs and whatever job we put him down for – even if he had asked for it the day before – he would not go to it when he came in.

We had a sign-in rule so that we knew who was on site, but when he came in late he would not tell anyone he had arrived and would start on a job he could see needed doing. Whatever he did was always useful. He was clearly conscientious and had thought about it, he just never discussed it with us or stuck to what he had asked to do the day before. It was very puzzling.

I went on a course on the Human Givens and first of all they asked us to rate ourselves on each of the categories. This was personally interesting and offered new insights. Then it was suggested you put yourself into the shoes of someone you found it difficult to work with or understand. I immediately chose Ian and tried to make the same choices through his eyes. He had been (and no doubt still was) a very skilled and successful therapist, highly thought of in his field. Although I found myself scoring him relatively low in many categories, the one that really hit rock bottom was social status. I suddenly understood that this man had lost all sense of his own worth. My exasperation and fear of tackling him just seemed to evaporate. The next day, I waited for him to come in and asked him to explain how he felt when he came in late and everyone had started without him. I also said that I felt we hadn't got it quite right for him and would like to do better, but that he might need to help us do so.

He became upset and the brittle facade collapsed. I was shocked by what he told me, perhaps because I was a bit in awe of his skill and reputation as a therapist. He said he came in late deliberately because he couldn't bear to have to start the day's job with other people, because they would see how stupid he was. So, he came in after everyone else had started and just got on with whatever he could see needed doing. Horrified that he should be so lacking in confidence, we made an agreement that when he came in, he should come and see me and I would then talk through the jobs on offer and could personally coach him through whatever it involved. It wasn't a quick fix, but we had opened a much more fruitful dialogue that led to some truly healing work on distressing issues from his past.

A SENSE OF MEANING IN LIFE AND A PURPOSE TO WHAT WE DO

What floats your boat? What gets you excited? What do you feel is important? What do you think would make the world a better place? What do you want to do?

When you are in the thick of mental health problems, recovery seems impossible, so you need something else that you really believe in to inspire you – to motivate you to make that enormous effort to get beyond your fears and anxieties. It needs to be something bigger than yourself, and something that you can commit to, believe in and really want to do, despite feeling low.

People coming to volunteer in a garden do not want to be useless; they do not want to be labelled 'victims' or 'patients, and hate the term 'service users' (which is much used in mental services and circles). Most of us feel excited to be part of building something that could change lives, and, in doing so, change our own.

FEELING STRETCHED AND STIMULATED

Many people describe being depressed and anxious as unbearably boring. They long for something to do; something with real meaning.

> I was once enlisted to deliver a weekly class on a horticultural theme to a group of elderly men living in a residential care home. Most of them were too frail to go outside and it was during the winter months, so they were all pretty much housebound. I decided to show them how to take cuttings of house plants and pot them up in the care home so they could learn to look after them.

On my first visit, I was shown into a carpeted living room where I was expected to work. Then I was shown the cupboard where the last adult education worker had kept her materials. As I open the cupboard door, a load of small woollen dolls fell out. This was apparently the last 'meaningful activity' these men had been involved with. I went back to the living room with my pots and plants and compost, switched off the blaring television which was broadcasting *Playschool*, and we proceeded to have a great time making lots of mess. Many of them soon remembered that they knew lots about gardening.

In one garden, for some reason, we seemed to attract very highly qualified and skilled people; usually, half the volunteers on site had at least one university degree. They often enjoyed and needed complex tasks to keep them interested. This could prove challenging. If a volunteer is undertaking a complicated project and becomes unwell for a time, it can be hard for the staff to take over the reins. We had to encourage people to teach us as they went along and to take copious notes for us.

When I was attending another training seminar on 'human givens', Joe Griffin, the lecturer and author of *Human Givens*,[33] told a story to illustrate how an understanding of this structure could help you work effectively with someone, without having to know much about their history. You just needed to know where they are now. In the way stories do, it has stuck with me for over twenty years.

One day, the local minister was reminded that he hadn't seen Mrs Jones in church for many months. It was coming up to the anniversary of her husband's death – they had been married for over fifty years and she was an elderly lady. Before she lost her husband, she had been a regular attendee of the church and supported many of its groups. He realised he had maybe been a bit remiss in not offering her more support, so he decided to go and visit her. She was at home and although she welcomed him in, her mood seemed flat and low. He quickly ascertained that she seldom went out or indeed saw any of her old friends or neighbours. She seemed to have withdrawn inside herself.

He was hunting around trying to raise a flicker of interest in her when he noticed some attractive flowering plants on several of the windowsills. He asked her what they were called, commenting on how lovely they were. She at once became more animated and, smiling for the first time, told him they were African Violets. He asked if they had been a gift from someone, but she said she propagated them herself from leaf cuttings. They talked a bit more about the plants and then he asked her if she had some to spare. She said she always had some to spare, that she struggled to find enough space for them on the windowsill. He then asked her if she would be willing to donate some to the church as he often had to visit people who were ill in hospital or hospices, and they would make lovely gifts. She said she would be delighted, and how many would he like, and that she could take lots more cuttings... And so began her way back into living, not just staying alive, and into achieving a much higher score on the Human Givens scale. She became the 'African Violet Lady' with a sense of belonging, feelings of self-worth, emotional connection to others, social status, meaning, and purpose.

PLAYFULNESS

Playfulness is often, though not always, lost when people become very depressed or anxious. Sometimes people are just too exhausted for various reasons connected to poor mental health. Sometimes they have just got out of the habit. Sometimes they have just never learnt the knack. On occasion, they are afraid to look as if they are enjoying themselves in case onlookers think they're not really feeling as bad as they have said they do.

The best support workers in a garden are also the most playful.

> I remember a time when some people were getting a bit tetchy and grumbling about having to do the daily cleaning duty. We had explained the need for everyone to pull their weight, how no one was exempt, but the grumbling continued and became a bit demoralising. One day, after a few weeks of this, one of the male staff – a big burly guy with long, curly blond hair and the beginnings of a beard – turned up wearing a frock and a big frilly pinny, his long hair fluffed up, with a cigarette hanging out of his mouth. He was carrying a bucket and mop and he got to work cleaning the floor. He totally broke the mood as everyone fell about laughing and then got into gear.

Other volunteers always make my day better with their great sense of humour and witty one-liners. Some have gone to great lengths with jokes and play acting to brighten up the days for the rest of us.

To this end, it's great to have lots of bonfires, tea parties, little treats, jokes, snowmen and sledging, spontaneous walks along the river and trips to the seaside, just because you can.

2. *THE TIDAL MODEL*[34] BY PHIL BARKER AND POPPY BUCHANAN-BARKER AND THEIR COLLEAGUES

Gardening doesn't always go to plan. Sometimes the potatoes get blight. Heavy winds can blow down and damage trees. In one of the community gardens where I work, a deer once came in and systematically nibbled all the flower buds of every single godetia plant. You have to see this in the perspective of being part of the natural world, where we don't always have control. It will have its ups and downs, good seasons and bad, just like sailing on a long voyage. It's not a reason to give up. In fact, those plants came back stronger and, because of their unplanned pruning, they were bushier and had more flowers than ever.

This is a philosophical approach to the discovery of mental health, using the metaphor of the voyage.

It can be hard for people to articulate their feelings, especially when they try to talk about the most powerful emotions, such as grief after a bereavement, or the joy of a new birth. To explain our feelings we often reach into our imagination to use similes and metaphors to illustrate what these experiences mean to us. I learnt from listening to the inspirational Phil and Poppy Barker about the Tidal Model metaphor, described on their website:

Life is a voyage undertaken on an ocean of experience.
All human development, including the experience of illness
and health, involves discoveries made on that voyage.
At critical points in the voyage the person may experience
storms or even piracy – in everyday terms this might be
*called a **crisis**.*
At other times the ship may begin to take in water and the
person may face the prospect of drowning or shipwreck –
*commonly called a **breakdown**.*
The person may seek – or be guided to – a safe haven, to

undertake repairs, or otherwise address the effects of the
*trauma – we might call this **rehabilitation**.*
 Only once the ship is made intact, and the person has
regained the necessary sea-legs, can the ship set sail again,
aiming to put the person back on the life course.
*This is the next stage in the **voyage of recovery**.*[35]

I like *The Tidal Model* for its insights into what is going
wrong with some of our mental health service practices. We all
take them for granted but they could be done differently.

It encourages giving feedback in the form of small incremental changes. When someone is in extreme distress, a
perceived small improvement, such as someone talking a bit
more, being able to look up at me briefly, able to weep, able to
drink a cup of tea in company, are all significant. As someone
returns from a state of numbness, they may feel worse rather
than better, as they are reconnecting with emotions that may
be overwhelming. However, from the outside, we might be
able to give feedback on this and celebrate it as an improvement. Giving witness to someone really helps them to begin to
understand what progress might feel like, and that some real
movement is happening.

The Tidal Model also talks about people being governed by
commitments rather than commandments. If people's values
and commitments are right, good practice will follow. Do I
treat people the way that I would want people to treat me or
my loved ones if they became unwell or distressed? It goes on
to describe ten commitments (taken from the book *The Tidal
Model* by Phil Barker and Poppy Buchanan-Barker):

- The voice – encourage the person's true voice
  rather than enforce the voice of authority

211

- Respect the language – respect the person's own way of telling the story, don't interpret

- Become the apprentice – the person is the expert on their story. Be the learner

- Use the available toolkit – what does the person believe has worked or might work?

- Craft the step beyond – work together to discover what needs to be done now/ what is the first step to take on the road to recovery

- The gift of time – in supporting people, it's our time that makes the difference

- Develop genuine curiosity – try to help the person tell you their story. You need to have some understanding of the whole story not just signs and symptoms of disease. It might be something completely unrelated to their distress that points the way to recovery, e.g. a love of music/nature/art

- Know change is constant – nothing lasts. Help the person become aware of the nature of change and how they could make a decision that affects what they will do next to bring about their recovery

- Reveal personal wisdom – people have usually learnt what works for them but might need help to remember

- Be transparent with others – become a team

The book *The Tidal Model* and the website are both very accessible and easy to follow.

3. *LANGUISHING TO FLOURISHING*[36] BY COREY KEYES – A SOCIAL MODEL OF RECOVERY

Keeping a plant alive is not the be all and end all. You can keep that acid loving azalea alive in a lime-rich part of the garden – perhaps you wanted it to grow in front of an old garden wall that is lime rendered and has been leaching into the soil over many years? However, it will only be alive, not well and flourishing, and you will never see its glorious potential. It won't make your heart sing. If you find out what it really wants and needs and you move it to a new situation where the soil is more acid, it might not be exactly where you wanted it to be, but you will see it flourish.

Corey Keyes, a Canadian social psychologist, researches the rise of depression in the twentieth century, and the converging fall in our sense of community belonging. He is interested in the way of thinking that starts with 'I feel', the way of thinking that puts the individual right at the centre of everything that is happening, as opposed to what is happening in the community.

A post on the blog Return to Now refers to an aboriginal Australian saying that in his language, there are no words directly translating as 'mine' or 'yours', but instead the culture emphasises our place in a social community:

While modern parents force … children to say 'please' and 'thank you', Aborigines find the words offensive, as they imply ownership and are seen as 'begging'. Like most hunter-gatherers, they have no concept of private property and treat fellow tribe members literally as extensions of themselves.

"In our language we have no such word as 'please' or 'thank you,' because it is expected of us that we share and give what we have," the man says. Hunter-gatherers have no concept of private property, so: "In the old days, it was a given that we would share. That was a part of who we are. Not only for aboriginal people – I expect people all around the world would do the same before money.

But nowadays we say 'it's mine!' There are words like 'mine' … We deny other people shelter, we deny other people food, we deny other people their survival purely because of money… and it kills us as human beings." [37]

My own father was born in 1911. He lived through two world wars and he had epilepsy in a time when it was little understood and had to be kept secret or he wouldn't be employed. He lost his job every time he had a seizure. Consequently, the family was always on a low income and the spectre of unemployment was never far away. If you had asked him how he felt about his life, if he was happy, he would not have known what you were talking about.

If you asked him to describe himself, he would probably have said he was a family man with four children, a strong union man, and a member of a political party. His social life revolved round his children, his brothers and sisters, and their families. He would never have made a statement beginning with "I feel". For him, life would be seen in terms of the strong community he lived in and, despite having an extremely hard life, he woke up singing every morning and went to work, glad to have any job at all, even if it was one well below his capabilities. He had a smile and a word for everyone he met on the street. The only time this changed was when he was out of a job, which was never for long.

If you think back to the Human Givens, he felt safe in the knowledge that his family and neighbours were all around him. He had a strong sense of belonging and purpose; his status was wrapped up in his family, his union activities and his politics. Despite the hardships he endured in his life, I would say that he flourished.

A recent piece of research by Sue Pinkerton[38] into longevity discovered the ten most important features contributing to a long life.

1. Having three close friends – people you can call in the middle of the night, borrow money from, go and stay with if you have to

2. Having many social relationships – talk to the man in the newsagents, your neighbours, and the postie; volunteer somewhere, join social groups

3 – 10. All the things you might have guessed at, including looking after your weight, blood pressure, diet, exercise, alcohol, and cigarette and drug consumption

Being part of a socially active community is good for you: it helps you to not just live longer but to flourish.

The biggest therapeutic influence of being involved with the garden was being part of something; belonging somewhere and having a sense of purpose. Many people were discharged from hospital when their symptoms appeared to be under control, usually through medication. For example, when they were not hearing voices anymore, not have psychotic episodes, not feeling suicidal, and not having rapid mood swings. While all of that might be helpful to someone, in itself it is just living and not the same as having a fulfilled life. To flourish, people need to be involved in something that excites them and makes them want to get up in the morning, and this can happen despite symptoms of mental ill health.

4. CREATING A SAFE SPACE

I once worked in an old Victorian greenhouse which looked beautiful and well-constructed on the outside, but the plants simply did not thrive in it. There were always problems with pests and disorders. The light was wrong, the watering system was inadequate, the airflow wasn't right. It took a long time to work out why the conditions were wrong and what would turn this into a healthy growing space.

Feeling emotionally safe is important to all of us but never more so than when someone, especially someone with a history of trauma, feels vulnerable and afraid; then it is the most important thing of all. How you go about creating that feeling of being in a safe place is seldom talked about in any project or service description. Terms or jargon which don't actually have a common agreed meaning, such as 'respect' and 'confidentiality', 'involvement' and 'empowerment', are used, as if we already have an understanding of what they mean and know how they are achieved.

This use of language ignores context and doesn't explain any details or methods. Does 'confidential' mean I will never disclose what you tell me, or that I will only disclose it to my supervisor, or that I will only disclose it to the staff team? Will it be written in a file, and if so, who can read that, and under what circumstances? If I am worried about your safety, will I call the emergency services? It can make something that is neb-ulous or fuzzy seem stable, mechanical and precisely defined when actually I have found this to be far from the case. People have their own, very individual definitions of all these terms. In the particular example of confidentiality, it is important to make sure people understand what confidentiality will mean in the garden group context. Before people confide in you, they need to know what to expect.

It is a constant challenge to make a project or service involv-ing a large group of people feel safe. What does that mean?

There are lots of subgroups of the feeling of safety:

- Do the volunteers feel safe with each other?

- Do the volunteers feel safe with the staff?

- Do members of the public feel safe?

- Do the staff team feel safe with each other, the volunteer group, and with the manager?

- Do people feel safe within the line management structure of the company?

- Do people feel safe working for that company?

In order to feel safe, people need to feel listened to, to be as relaxed as is possible for them, and to be able to voice their opinions honestly without worrying about displeasing you.

Ask people what works for them. Would you rather wait by yourself or in the canteen with the others? Would you rather talk in my office or in the garden? Would you rather sit in the garden or go for a walk? People usually feel safer when they have choices. Oddly, many agencies that should know better seldom allow such choices.

An atmosphere of decency, openness and friendliness between everyone involved, no matter what their role, is essential for people to thrive. It is the basis for healthy, therapeutic outcomes for everyone.

Staff need to be careful not to get too hung up on 'being the professional' and letting rules and a bureaucracy get in the way of honest human connection. I found the idea of 'coming from a clean place' i.e. one that puts the other person's welfare first, and not getting hijacked by your own needs, really helpful.

Everyone has bad days. Everyone needs to be able to flag them up and receive support. You could be having a long and tiring day, with seven hours of hard, physical work, and at the same time be managing groups of people, some of whom are upset and need a lot of support. If you are not on form, your team need to know so they can look out for you.

5. RESPONDING CREATIVELY TO PROBLEMS AT THE TIME

If you find greenfly on your tomatoes or slugs attacking your courgettes, then you need to deal with them straight away. A wait-and-see approach is not likely to bring about the change you need save your crops

If you see something that does not feel right, someone's behaviour for instance, some comment or statement, or a lack of consultation, then it helps to present it to the group as a series of facts rather than as an emotional story about how you feel. It is also better if it is presented in a timely fashion and not months after the event. Always make sure you offer a positive suggestion for what would have worked better for you.

I noticed that Jim had spoken several times about the paid members of staff at the large community garden where he worked. He felt that they seemed to forget sometimes that the volunteers were part of the team.

In general, he liked all of the staff and volunteers, and got on well with them. The members of staff only worked part time hours in the garden and Jim worked many more. He was also a very experienced gardener, probably more so than the members of staff, and had been involved in the garden for much longer.

It seemed to him that when anything happened in the garden that was newsworthy, it was always the members of staff who talked to the press and were in the photo shoots for the papers, even when volunteers were in attendance and available. Also, fairly major decisions were made without consultation with the volunteer gardeners, many of whom had experience in management as well as gardening. Often, things which had been agreed in consultation with the volunteers in the past would be changed by the new staff members with no warning.

I actually think that the members of staff would be quite horrified if they knew how he was feeling, as they are very committed to their work in the garden. If Jim had been able to address each issue as it came up, not in a blaming way but by offering a factual report of what he observed and how it could have been handled differently, it would probably have been well received, and indeed they might have very good reasons for their behaviour that Jim was not aware of. Offering suggestions helps individuals feel more involved and it achieves results, rather than allowing them to carry on feeling disgruntled, which may result in them leaving the group.

I have heard similar versions of Jim's story from other people on quite a few occasions, and from different garden projects.

6. RESPONDING TO CRITICISM POSITIVELY

This can be particularly difficult for people with responsibility. On one hand, they feel they need to be seen as people with some authority, but at the same time, they are held accountable and are expected to be able to discuss their actions and words with whoever questions them.

Thankfully, I have been fortunate to have worked in gardens where other members of staff felt comfortable to question my judgement. These people weren't having a go at me, they had my back.

Similarly, "Oh I was only joking" kind of horseplay and teasing cannot be encouraged. There is a difference between playful teasing and cruel teasing, and most people, even if they are quite unwell, can recognise that difference straight away. It's important to deal with disputes and disagreements openly, and lay differences on the table for discussion.

Respect a complaint. It takes courage to confront perceived authority. For someone who has lived the disempowering label of 'mental health service user', making a complaint can be seen as a huge success, not a failure. Sensitive discussions lead to valuable insight and learning.

7. BATHE[39] – AN ACRONYM FOR A FAST FIRST RESPONSE

Every garden should have a first aid kit. You are unlikely to have the resources to solve any major injury, but with the right first aid kit and emergency first aid training, you will be able to help significantly. At the very least, you will be able to stop the injury getting worse and steer the individual towards appropriate help.

Anyone who works with people will know that sinking feeling when someone who is clearly upset wants to speak to you, but you only have half an hour to give them. I found this little format for working with that situation really helpful. It's called BATHE:

B – Background. Ask the person what has happened. They will want to tell you all the details and lots of complicated backstory, like who is who and relationships, etc. At this point, they probably believe that the more of the story they give you, the better you will be able to help them. Actually, you really only need to know the bare bones. The details might help them in the telling but they won't assist you in the understanding or in your ability to help. After five minutes, you will probably have the gist and should try to gently move the discussion on to the next stage.

A – How have you been **affected** by what has happened? (Unable to sleep, not eating enough, overeating, drinking too much, isolating myself, feeling anxious, worrying about everything, and so on.) Again, five minutes is long enough, as all you are trying to do is get them thinking a bit more analytically. So, move on to the next stage.

T – What is the most **traumatic** aspect of what has happened? With a little encouragement, people will usually be able to identify the worst part of the problem for them. By now, they may be back in thinking mode and can begin to work things out, so focus on what is upsetting them the most.

H – What **helps**? People are the experts on themselves. You cannot know enough to help someone in half an hour, but they will have their own insights if you encourage them to think about it. Have you felt like this before? What helped then? (I phoned my sister, I went to see my doctor, I went to my yoga class again, I used to like drawing...) Gradually, revisiting what helped in the past will start to nudge the person into using the more rational and problem-solving part of their brain. They should feel more positive that they have survived a similar circumstance before and might be able to do so again. Now, between you, you can come up with a short-term plan, perhaps to just get them through the weekend, based on what they know has helped them before. You have probably used up your half hour by now, but don't forget the last stage.

E – **Empathy:** "I am so sorry this has happened to you and is making you feel so bad; I hope you feel a bit better soon. I'm glad you told me about it, we can talk more next week."

8. BUILDING EMOTIONAL MUSCLE

Two of the gardens I work in are located on steep slopes. When volunteers first start, they often struggle to walk up to the top of the garden. It's truly amazing how quickly this changes. No matter where people start, they end up getting fitter and by the end of the summer they can walk up and down the hill without giving it much thought. They just have to start.

Most people understand that if you want to be an athlete or a body builder you are going to have to spend a regular amount of time in the gym. People don't always find it easy to accept that building emotional muscle requires exactly the same effort and commitment. It's a process of challenging long and deeply-held beliefs about yourself, such as, 'nobody wants me here, I am useless, it would be better for everyone if I was gone…' The only way to overcome such beliefs and feelings is to constantly challenge them. This is best done with help from someone who can give an honest outside opinion.

A typical exercise I might give someone would be something like: "When you come in in the morning, look up at the first person you meet and say 'hello'. If they say hello back then ask them something like, 'What are you working on today?' and then report back to me."

The response will usually be "Yes, they said hello" and "Yes, they were happy to talk to me."

Or maybe I will ask them to write down three good things that happened to them each day, no matter how small e.g. "I heard the birds singing on the way in", "Jane said I had made a good job of planting the potatoes", "One of my neighbours nodded to me on the way to the garden." These little happenings build up a body of proof that people actually seem to like and value them, and that offers little glimmers of light. People often find this simple exercise excruciatingly hard to do. It's as if they don't believe that the two things can coexist – their feelings of depression and abject misery, and good things happening to them, however small. People also express the worry that has been mentioned before, that if they talk about good things happening others may stop believing they feel as low as they do.

Daily exercises and regular practice when you are not in the worst moments of distress can do wonders to help you manage difficult situations when they arise. If you wait till a panic attack happens before enacting positive behaviours, then your brain won't be working well enough to give you much help. But if you work daily on exercises to reduce tension and anxiety, then you might not end up having panic attacks at all, or at the very least they will be less severe.

There are numerous self-help books like the popular *Feel the Fear and Do It Anyway*[40] by Susan Jeffers, and websites like Moodgym[41] which are also helpful. Other people use yoga, meditation, tai chi, walking – anything that you find relaxes you and calms your system. But whatever it is, it needs to be done regularly to become a daily habit. As one of my friends often says to people, "don't just drop in on your mental health."

9. WORKING WITH CHANGE

We all get attached to our gardens, but then life gets in the way. When I was a young mother with two small children, feeling rooted was very important to me. We had to move house five times within three years and each time I hated leaving the garden I had just painstakingly created. I could take some of the smaller plants with me. My garden plants often have quite a sentimental attachment for me: maybe gifted by friends, or the crocuses I regularly took to my mother in her last days in hospital. After some sadness at having to leave plants behind, I learnt to plan for the day I had to move and took cuttings of all the plants I had a special soft spot for. If it turned out I didn't need them, they made nice presents for friends or donations for plant sales.

In one garden, we used to work with a group with learning disabilities who ran a catering service in town. When they cleared out their freezers to put in fresh stock, they used to donate some of the produce to the garden for our volunteers to have. This was a kindness we appreciated very much, as it was excellent quality food and our volunteers were nearly all on very low budgets. As a thank you, we offered the use of the garden to that group and their families for a party to be held one Sunday in summer, when it was normally closed to the public.

All the plans were made for food and entertainment, and we were expecting around fifty guests. Just because I was in the office, I decided to check my emails about an hour before people were due to arrive and found an email saying that the insurance had changed and that no external groups were allowed to use the garden unless the new forms had been filled in and agreed by management! No management people were in the office because it was the weekend. Total panic ensued.

The team, myself included, were raging and huffing and puffing about what a disaster this was, when the one member of the team who was not moaning and groaning with us came out of the office and said he had arranged for a church up the road to let us use their hall and garden. All we had to do was shift the catering supplies and meet people at the top of the drive and redirect them just a quarter of a mile to the new venue. It all worked, and everyone had a great time. While we were all grumbling about our changed situation, he had not wasted any time and had gone straight into 'sort it' mode.

I had this clear moment of realisation about how much time I had wasted in my life bemoaning and mourning changes that

I could do nothing about, instead of moving on and working out how I could manage them. It was such a valuable lesson.

Of course, people need time to mourn any serious losses in their life, but a good understanding of how we manage change is invaluable. I came across this little book, *Who Moved My Cheese?* by Spencer Johnson,[42] which I really like and found helpful. We live in a transient and fast-changing world, and to get too attached to what is, without ever pondering what if or what might be, can make life very difficult to manage. I believe I now value my cheese much more in the knowledge that it is unlikely to last forever, and I also try to keep options for 'what if' in my mind too.

It is understandable that people are afraid of change – better the devil you know, and all of that – but it is good to introduce the notion that without change we are all stuck exactly where we are. If that is depressed or anxious, then change is the only way forward, however scary it might feel.

10. THE BLACK DOG – DEPRESSION LIES TO YOU

In a bad year when the weather is foul, yields are low, diseases and pests are on the rampage, it can be hard to stay positive, especially in the veg garden. I find it helpful to visit other gardens and speak to the people there about what's going on. Have they had a bad season too? Have they discovered a better system of growing anything that I could learn from? It's good to do something and not just brood on things and get discouraged. Try to focus on what has grown well.

Depression lies to you. It tells you, "Stay home today, don't go out. Just stay in bed, it's much safer, only bad things will happen if you go out and meet people. You will fail at anything you try to do today". What it doesn't tell you is that if you stay in bed today it will be there under the covers with you all day, dripping its poison into your ear.

Depression lies to you.

I love the little books written by Matthew Johnstone. *I Had a Black Dog, His Name Was Depression*[43] is a cartoon book which describes what it feels like to have depression and how to begin to deal with it. It's a beautiful, sensitive, and actually quite funny book, and people with depression always say, "That's me. That's how I feel" when you give it to them. There is a similar partner book called *Living with the Black Dog*, which is for people who are trying to support someone with depression. These are great books to have lying around in waiting rooms and on coffee tables.

11. UNDERSTANDING NEGATIVE SELF-TALK

I often work with volunteers who are a bit older and who have been very successful in their careers. They are used to being good at what they do and if they have not learnt about gardening before, they can feel very deskilled when they first arrive. They may have had their own garden and tried to grow things unsuccessfully, perhaps many times over, so they have come to think of themselves as 'useless' gardeners. These people will often come to the community garden saying they simply don't have green fingers and that they will stick to clearing the paths. They tend to do much better working alongside people with more experience of growing things in the garden, who can show them what to do. Although any success is a shared outcome, it is also a positive one.

We all have an inner dialogue running in our heads that influences our mood, how we feel about ourselves, and our subconscious decision making. This is not the same as hearing voices but can be a bit similar in effect and influence. One of the big differences is that people are usually very aware of the voices they hear but are often not, or much less, aware of their inner dialogue.

The first step in awareness is to listen out for trigger words in your thought streams. At one point in my life, I was driving 30 miles each way to work and spending all day in the garden working hard physically. This involved supporting people with severe and enduring mental health problems. I was also bringing up two children. My mother had died not long before and I missed her terribly, although I was fortunate to have a very supportive partner.

> When we began to look at negative self-talk and its effects on people and ourselves, I tried to tune in more to what was going on in my head as I drove home. I noticed that the word tired kept occurring: "Oh I feel so tired/ exhausted/knackered. Tonight, I'm looking forward to just sitting in front of the fire" and similar moans. Then I would get home and often do just that. But sometimes, a friend would come round and ask if we wanted to go for a cycle, run, walk, or to a music session in the pub. Before my negative thoughts kicked in, I would be at the door saying, "Sounds great, let's go."

I wasn't really that tired at all: it was just a habitual frame of mind. People were always reinforcing this by saying to me, "Oh I don't know how you manage that driving every day." Truth be told, I loved it. Not only was it necessary to put some distance between my work and my children, it was two hours of the day which I got entirely to myself on a lovely rural road with little traffic. I had my mug of tea and my story tape and was happy as anything.

I learnt to listen for the tired talk in my head so I could interrupt it. I would physically hit the steering wheel or ping the elastic band I wore on my wrist and say out loud, "No I'm not" and switch to a more positive thought pattern, sing a song, turn on the radio or an audiobook, plan a holiday, and find some way to stop it in its tracks.

The interesting thing about positive self-talk is that you don't need to believe it for it to work. Our brain works like a computer and will believe what you tell it. So if you are programmed by others during a toxic childhood to believe that you are stupid, ugly and useless (all of which are trigger words), and you reinforce this every day with your own negative self-talk along the same lines, then your brain will believe it, even though the rest of the world can see you are attractive, clever, kind and highly-skilled in many areas. I came to believe that this contrast between what someone believes about themselves and how others see them is almost a defining symptom of trauma.

It can be difficult for people with this experience to say anything positive about themselves at all, and sometimes the 'good enough' compromise works better at least to start with.

It's not, of course a quick fix. If someone has been telling themselves negative things for thirty-plus years, it's going to take a while to reprogram the brain, as well as lots of feedback from others until they can do it for themselves. They need to learn to recognise when they are talking to themselves negatively, and actively look for ways to reframe their thoughts.

Gordon had been horribly bullied at school. He was small and slight of build and the bigger lads had made his life an absolute misery. He was an extremely skilled craftsman and could do just about anything with his hands. He would be building things in the garden like seed boxes and would have produced ten perfectly already, but when he made a small mistake on the eleventh one. He would let out an absolute torrent of abuse against himself that bore no relation to his achievements.

He had become so used to the slagging he had received, that he had become his own bully. We had to work with him for a long time to help him see his achievements and to persuade him we did not believe any of the truly awful insults he hurled at himself. It helped to try to make him think about how he would talk to someone else who had made the same mistake. Would he shout at them like he did to himself? "Of course not," he would say, "They couldn't help it; they were doing their best." And slowly, with much repetition, we would establish a policy of 'same rules' for everybody, including himself.

12. UNDERSTANDING, TOLERATING AND MANAGING SELF-HARM

In the years after my back injury, I knew that I needed exercise and that I needed to be in the garden working, but there were still things that could trigger a bad back episode. The most common one was digging. Despite using a small border fork and knowing I needed to pace myself, I would often get too caught up in the task. Wanting to do it myself, I would overdo it and damage my back and so end up in a lot of pain for the following weeks. There was a fine line between getting exercise and harming myself.

Working with self-harm can be very frightening and unsettling for everyone, especially if it's severe and potentially life threatening. It's a very natural feeling to just want the person to stop. Sadly, that's not usually a very effective tactic.

Of course, we all self-harm to some extent. A couple of coffees a day won't harm you but eight or more probably does. A few glasses of wine at the weekend will probably do no harm but two bottles a night might. The occasional bar of chocolate or slice of cake won't hurt, but a daily helping might be bad for you. Cigarettes are known to be highly toxic, yet many indulge in this habit. Even exercise, which we generally think of as good for us, can be harmful if taken to excess. It's worth spending some time reading about this complex issue to try to get a better understanding of the causes, and to work towards successful treatment.

Many people have told me self-harm helps them to feel real and present when past memories of trauma are making them feel numb. This numbness makes them afraid they might just disappear, or that they will do something they can't recover from. For some, the pain helps give them a focus when memories feel too difficult to live with. Some people say that this pain feels like something they have control over when everything else feels beyond their control.

Sometimes, it seems to offer a way of telling the person's story, if that story included pain, disgust and humiliation, as it often did. Self-harming can be a visible record of how people feel about themselves and what has happened to them.

It's worth remembering that self-harm may be a person's way of dealing with unbearable feelings.

Alex came into the garden once with a wound on his leg so severe he had to show it to me, as he was in such pain

THE GARDEN CURE

he couldn't work. There was a lot of old scarring round the site on his skin, so it clearly wasn't the first time. I commiserated that it looked very painful and said that we should put a dressing on it to keep it clean. He started to weep and said that no one had ever said that to him before. On some occasions, when the wound had got badly infected, he had to go to hospital for treatment. He dreaded it, as he felt so ashamed of what he had done and thought that the staff would think his self-inflicted wounds would take time away from 'real' patients, and that he was just attention seeking.

Some people are able to use various tricks to cheat the feeling, like using a red pen to write on their arm instead of a knife or using an ice cube to cause pain instead of burning. A self-inflicted wound is every bit as painful as one received by accident.

13. THE RESCUE TRIANGLE[44] – UNDERSTANDING THE ROLES OF VICTIM, BULLY AND RESCUER

Plants can be bullies too. The wonderful mint that we all love in tea or on our new potatoes can quickly get out of hand and swamp the delicious, if somewhat less robust, parsley that we want to put in our soup. We need to keep a constant watch on our plants to make sure they stick to their boundaries.

In the rescue triangle, people can adopt the roles of victim, rescuer, and persecutor/bully, and can change roles within the relationship as it develops. Some people are particularly susceptible to being rescuers. They want to be the one who helps. It makes them feel good to do that. This is OK, so long as it is not at the expense of keeping the other person in a position of helplessness and causing them to become entrenched in the role of victim. By becoming dependant on the rescuer to save them each time, the 'victim' doesn't get the chance to develop any resilience. Clearly there is no growth in that, and the victim retains feelings of helplessness and being unable to cope alone.

The victim persona can switch to being the persecutor when they don't get the kind of "I'll sort it for you" support that they want from their rescuer; they can turn on the rescuer with an "It's all your fault" attitude of blame. Or it can happen the other way around; the rescuer loses patience if the victim doesn't accept the help being offered, and the rescuer can turn persecutor.

It's a fascinating way of looking at the role of the supporter and the person being supported. This model merits real consideration.

I once got trapped (oops, gone into victim mode already) into calling a man several times one evening because I was so worried about him. He had had a bad day (he was a potential suicide risk) and I agreed to call him when he got home (back from hospital) to make sure he was all right. I did so and then agreed to call again at bedtime. I still wasn't feeling confident and agreed to call him first thing in the morning. We did this for a couple of days. He was OK but I soon realised that I couldn't go on like that. I was undermining his confidence in his ability to keep himself safe. The more I called, the more I did just that, and I was beginning to feel like another victim of his anxiety. We then proceeded to work on what he could do for himself if he didn't feel safe, such as distraction techniques, friends he could call, helplines he could use and so forth.

14. PATTERNED BEHAVIOUR – HOW OUR BELIEFS AND BEHAVIOURS ARE FORMED

One of the issues that can arise in a community garden is gender stereotyping. I am female and little over 5'2. I was once offered a gardening job through correspondence. I signed myself J. Cameron. When I turned up on site, the owner took one look at me and instead of showing me into the walled garden, took me to the house and said there would be work for me in there with his mother. In groups of volunteers, men will often offer, with best intentions, to take over the sawing of a tree or building a bonfire from a woman, believing she will appreciate his help. Sometimes, the woman does not take kindly to what was a genuine offer of help and sees it instead as a slight on her capability. Different perceptions of roles can lead to discord. It works both ways of course. Women may assume that because a man looks bigger and stronger than she is, he will want to do the harder, more physical jobs all day, when in fact he has a bad back and would prefer to work in the greenhouse, thinning out seedlings.

We are creatures who learn by pattern matching. Our brain creates a system of overlays, which gradually build up our understanding of the world and how it works. For example, in very simple terms, if you had kind and loving parents, you are more likely to believe that people will be kind to you. If you had abusive parents, then it's unlikely you will be able to trust people easily. If you have experienced bad teachers at school, you are unlikely to want to go into further education because of that bad experience. So, our beliefs are made up from our experiences.

I have sometimes had problems with people who had had bad experiences at work with their line managers or bosses. They would cast me in the role of the demanding, critical and punitive boss, which I hope I never was. As I approached the group they were working with, they would make a great show of working hard. They would make comments like, "The boss is coming, look busy", etc. The other, longer-term volunteers found it quite amusing, but I found it wearing. It often took a long time to reshape their expectations of 'the boss'. For some of the men, it was especially tricky because I was a woman.

> Fiona had grown up in a very gender stereotyped institutional environment and believed that women should work in the kitchen and do laundry while the men worked outside in construction or gardening. She used to get genuinely upset when I went to go to work alongside the men in the garden. She would keep asking me to come and help make tea and so on, saying that the men could manage the work by themselves.

We all fall into these patterned ways of behaving. It can be really useful to look at what those patterns are and whether they are helpful.

15. DIALOGUING – HOW TO REACH PEOPLE WHO ARE OVERWHELMED WITH EMOTION

Gardens – especially those worked on by large groups of people – usually function better with clearly defined sections, borders, and good labelling and signage. Then everyone knows what is happening and where things are meant to be and to go. This is especially relevant when working with someone who may be feeling too intimidated to ask.

Dialoguing is a useful technique, which was used in a residential unit for emotionally distressed children where I worked. If a child was in a temper and out of control, it was usually impossible to talk to them at that point, but it was possible to talk through their behaviour with another member of staff within his hearing. Most of us can't resist listening in to what is being said about us, so it usually captured their attention. It helped to explain to the child what was going on and brought their temper down to a level that was more negotiable. It might go a bit like this:

> **Adult 1**:"John is really upset because he wants to watch the TV but it's time for dinner and I've have said it must go off."

> **Adult 2**:"I can understand why he might be upset by that, if he is watching something special."

> **Adult 1**:"Yes I agree, but John was warned that it would go off at dinnertime and he agreed to it at the start."

> **Adult 2**:"Maybe we could record the rest of the programme and John could watch it later on?"

> **John**:"It's fish fingers for dinner and I hate them! Can I have something else?"

In the garden, we would use a form of dialoguing to make sure we understood what was happening for someone and also to make it clear that, as critical information was shared between the support staff, a member of staff could not promise not to tell anyone. It might go bit like this:

> I would notice that Mary, a staff member, had been talking to Andrea in the garden for half an hour and that Andrea appeared to be very upset. I would take over some cups of tea and say:"I've noticed that you've been talking for a while

and thought you might like a drink. Andrea seems upset, was there anything I could do to help?"

Mary might say: "Yes, Andrea is very upset. Andrea would you mind if I just fill Jan in briefly with what you have been telling me? Please stop me if I get it wrong or if you want to add something."

Mary would then give me a brief account of what they had been talking about. It seemed to help people to hear their story told in a short and logical way, and often they would be able to add something or clarify something in a more logical and less emotionally distressed way.

It reinforced that, as a staff team, we would share information. It also made it clear that if Mary was not in the garden tomorrow or was busy, then I would know what was happening and Andrea could also come and talk to me. As a staff team who were responsible for supervising groups of people in a working garden, it was important that we could be interchangeable and swap with each other sometimes.

16. THE USE OF IMAGINATION

Ordering seeds and planning for next year in the garden is all about imagination. Why would we bother if we didn't stop and have a wee daydream about how beautiful things might look, how delicious vegetables might taste, how beguiling flowers might smell?

When you introduce the idea of visualisation to many people, they will say they don't have any imagination and can't do it. These will be the same people who rehearse every night how awful the next day is going to be.

Without realising it, some people work really well with imagery. They will often imagine how bad a future event is going to be, how stupid they are going to feel, and that there is no chance that anything good will happen. Of course, because they rehearse it so successfully every night, they are almost hard-wired to make it happen. Teaching visualisation techniques can help people rehearse things like being calm when they talk to a difficult person who belittles them, surviving a bus journey that usually causes them to panic, managing to stay in the supermarket queue when it's busy. There is considerable evidence from sports performance coaches that mental preparation can be as strengthening as actually doing physical exercises. Similarly, rehearsing mental and emotional situations can build expectations of success and help to carve a new, more successful, groove in your nervous system

17. TOTEMS – OBJECTS IMBUED WITH MEANING, AND HOW THEY CAN HELP

Because I have always been a gardener and it's not safe to wear metal on your fingers or round your neck, I have never worn any jewellery. Many years ago, my daughter bought a crystal drop on a leather string – one for herself and one for me. She thought having a string instead of a sliver chain might make it more appealing to me, and it did. My other daughter now has one too. I wear it every day and it makes me feel close to them.

Once people get used to the garden and begin to trust the people there, they will start to feel safe. They are often fine while they are in the garden but as soon as they have been home for a wee while, all the old doubts and fears will come rolling back. Sometimes, it can help to give them a little object or totem of the garden to take home with them, such as a nice smooth stone or piece of wood, maybe a chestnut or a

238

pinecone, and to add a script to go with it. The principal of the school for distressed boys where I worked used to make everyone a set of wooden worry beads from wood gathered on the estate. There were four on the leather string and when you touched each bead in turn you were to remember: the place, the staff, the boys, and when you touched the fourth you were to remember, "I am a very special person."

18. THE OBSERVING SELF[45] – HOW TO BECOME MORE OBJECTIVE ABOUT YOUR FEELINGS

For the most part, we just head down to the garden and get stuck in, becoming engrossed in the day's task. Usually that's fine, but sometimes it's a good idea to take an hour or two to step back and take stock. I call these my chocolate teapot days. What is doing well? What needs attention? What hasn't done so well and needs to be rethought? Are the paths safe for your elderly auntie? Is there anywhere to sit in the shade? Imagine seeing the garden through the eyes of a first-time visitor and try to be objective. What are its strengths and weaknesses? Where is its potential growth?

The observing self is our ability as humans to step outside of ourselves and look at the situation we are in. You can probably see it most easily when a tricky situation suddenly seems funny and you can laugh at yourself. You are on the outside looking in.

You can sometimes help people get out of 'trance states', which occur when they are overwhelmed with emotion, by asking them to grade the feelings they are having, physically and mentally.

"How anxious are you feeling on a scale of 1 to 10?"

> Simply by doing this they have to remove themselves from the anxious state for a moment to look at it objectively. This alone can sometimes lower their anxiety level a little.
>
> You can also use metaphors and analogies to help people achieve the observing self.

During the course of my working life, I've presented talks and workshops at a range of conferences. I've always done this with a small group of volunteers helping me. I noticed that the people who really engaged while helping me develop training on mental health issues seemed to recover more quickly in terms of their own mood, confidence, and self-awareness. To deliver training with me, they had to spend quite a lot of time going over their own experiences and thinking about how they might use and present them to others, in order to give those people a better understanding of what a mental health problem can feel like. They had to consider their thoughts and feelings from the perspective of someone else. It obliges people to view their own story from a distance, which eventually seems to make it less painful and helps them process it into memory. It's a bit like saving a file on your computer that you can pull up only when you want to, rather than having it running open all the time.

19. MODELLING BEHAVIOUR – ACTING OUT THE BEHAVIOURS AND ACTIONS YOU ARE ADVOCATING

The garden responds well to order, planning, and tidy habits. Tools work best when cleaned, sharpened and stored systematically. Plants thrive better with good routines for watering and feeding, checking for pests and regular deadheading. The habits of good husbandry rub off and help people to understand the importance of maintaining routines for their own health and well-being

There were always some people in a garden who, while they take part in all the activities and work well, never seem to engage particularly with anyone, in that they don't ask for support or for time to talk about themselves. They just get on and work in the garden at whatever they are asked to do. They seldom engage much socially with the other volunteers but are perfectly pleasant to everyone. I think of them as 'observers'.

One such young man, Lenny, who had previously worked as a physiotherapist, came into my office one day after being with us for about eighteen months. He asked if he could talk to me, which was surprising, and said he felt it was time to leave. He was going to try and set up his practice again and he went on to thank me profusely for his time in the garden and all the help and support he had been given. I was taken aback. At that time, I felt we had not done very much for him. Even so, I wished him the best of luck and saw him on his way.

I thought a lot about it and began to realise that for some people *not* being asked lots of questions about their past, and *not* being made to engage in ways they didn't want to or weren't ready for, was just the kind of support they needed. He had been offered a safe space to take stock and work things out for himself. I realised that people like Lenny observe and absorb everything that is going on, like everything people say and the way they interact with each other. I realised, too, that it is important that we are aware that some people need the privacy and space to do things their own way. In the school where I worked, the staff might have called it 'role modelling'

– acting out positive, alternative ways of behaving that might differ from the behaviour the children experienced at home.

20. JOHN MUIR: "THE POWER OF THE IMAGINATION MAKES US INFINITE" – AN ECO-THERAPY MODEL

I love the recent movement of 'ungardening' – allowing part of your garden to go wild, letting nature have a space and offering habitat for insects and animals. I am not in the least upset to see the gradual demise of soldier rows of bedding plants surrounding manicured lawns in front gardens. It makes me sad to see so many people taking out their garden hedges, those absolute havens for wildlife, and replacing them with sterile walls.

John Muir was the pioneer of nature conservation. His is a fascinating life story and his influence in setting aside national parks changed how we think about nature and our role in protecting and preserving it. The John Muir Trust offers training in conservation leadership for people who work in gardens and the environment. Although it is recommended and very rewarding to do, you don't have to undertake the official leadership training in order to run a group for a John Muir award. However, some leadership skills and knowledge of working with groups in the environment are necessary. It is great fun and everyone I know who has taken part has loved it. A group can be anything that works: colleagues, friends, or a family. I did an award with my grandchildren one summer.

There are no exams or assignments in the John Muir Awards, as it only asks for commitment. You have to register your group with the John Muir Trust, and they will lead you through it. Then people just have to turn up and give it their best shot. There are four stages to each course – discovering, exploring, conserving, and sharing. Usually, groups of about eight people run one morning a week over three months.

POWER TOOLS

You can do lots of activities designed to help people appreciate their surroundings. My personal favourite is making potato rafts. You ask people to pair up, and give each pair a potato and a piece of string. They have to build a raft out of natural objects and float their potato on it. Then, they put them in the river and have a race. People are encouraged to keep a log of their days, either by writing things down, taking photographs, drawing, or whatever they want. To conserve the area, you can do litter picks, plant wildflowers to increase the biodiversity, take out invasive species, and build pathways. It's always good to have a bonfire; take turns to learn how to build one, then make tea and tell stories round the fire. Sharing can take the form of delivering a talk to the other people who aren't in the group, visual displays of photos, artwork, and a tour of the area and viewing of sculptures *in situ.*

For some people, the whole experience is fun and not too challenging. For others, it can take a long time to learn how to manage even four hours away from the garden even in a field just outside of it. It can be a real learning curve.

Everyone who completes the course gets a rather handsome certificate provided by the John Muir Trust. For some people, it might be the only certificate they have ever received. For others, it can be infinitely more valuable than their double first from Oxford.

Everybody needs beauty as well as bread, places to play and pray in, where nature may heal and give strength to body and soul.

John Muir

CHAPTER 15

THE BOOKSHELF

These resources might encourage you to look for a course, an experienced professional, or further study and training.

If you have a garden and a library, you have everything you need

Cicero

COURSES & TRAINING

1. NONVIOLENT COMMUNICATION[46]
Also known as Compassionate Communication, Nonviolent Communication is based on the principles of nonviolence coming from a state of compassion. It offers a course in how to communicate with compassion, using language structured to this end. I particularly enjoyed the small book on understanding 'The Surprising Purpose of Anger', which talks about seeing anger as the red light on the dashboard. It can be alarming, but it is not the thing to focus your attention on. You have to look under the bonnet to find out what is wrong. Courses are interactive and very accessible.

2. ALTERNATIVES TO VIOLENCE PROGRAMME (AVP)[47]
Described as 'a volunteer conflict transformation programme'. Teams of AVP facilitators conduct experiential workshops to develop a participant's ability to resolve conflicts without

resorting to manipulation, coercion, or violence. This is a group experience for anyone who wants to learn how to handle conflict, whether in the family, on the streets, in the workplace or somewhere else. Many of us in the garden team attended these weekend courses and we all gained a lot from the many scenarios and games used to help practice reactions and strategies. See website for more information, AVP workshops and courses near you. Courses are interactive and very accessible.

3. THE ALEXANDER TECHNIQUE[48]

The Alexander Technique, pioneered by FM Alexander in the late 1800s, provides a remarkable path to balanced, creative living. It is used worldwide by people from all walks of life. Through learning and applying the Technique it is possible to replace restrictive and painful postural habits with more effective patterns of movement accompanied by a fresh sense of lightness, freedom and well-being.

I am very fortunate to have been introduced to the Alexander Technique. It's about so much more than just correct posture. It gave me an insight into how to change the way I work with myself and other people. My teacher would ask me to do something, then she would most often say, "In a minute but not now", which kind of became my mantra for a while. Then we would be asked whether we wanted to do the action or not do it, or whether we wanted to do something completely different. It is a very different kind of teaching. I find myself fascinated by trying to discover that split-second moment in which I make choices. When I sit down at my computer, do I just sit in my usual habitual posture or do I stop to think about how I would like to be sitting? Do I need to rush down the stairs to answer the phone (as is my habit), or could I just walk down and either catch it in time or pick up the message and phone back? Or, could I choose to ignore it altogether if I need some time to myself? When I react to that difficult person speaking to me, do I react as I usually do, or do I find a moment to stop and reflect on how I would like to react? I'm still chasing that moment when I can make a choice and not just follow my habit, both physically and emotionally.

On her website, Alexander teacher Sarah Bonner-Morgan says of her work:

> *"The Technique teaches us the skilful "use of the self", i.e. how we use ourselves when moving, resting, breathing, learning, organising our awareness and focus of attention and, above all, choosing our reactions to increasingly demanding situations."*

4. SUICIDAL FEELINGS – ASIST TRAINING[49]

Working with people who are often plagued with suicidal thoughts is a large part of the work in therapeutic gardens, however it is now recognised as an ever-growing concern in our society. Over time, I came to learn the signs of someone feeling critically suicidal: the person coming to say goodbye at the end of the day when they don't usually, the person saying thank you for all the help you have given them before they go home. The most misleading of all is when someone who had previously been very anxious seems to develop a kind of euphoria, seeming to be suddenly calm and at peace, and also the person who suddenly, for no apparent reason, starts to give away all their belongings.

There is a growing need for suicide prevention training to be rolled out to the whole community and I thoroughly recommend taking part in the ASIST training (Applied Suicide Intervention Skills Training). These are two-day interactive workshops and anyone over the age of 16 can attend. Exactly like doing medical first aid training, you never know when you might be able to save someone's life.

LITERATURE

5. WORKING WITH TRAUMA

The Body Remembers,[50] *Babette Rothschild*
Help for the Helper,[51] *Babette Rothschild*
Waking the Tiger,[52] *Peter Levine*
In an Unspoken Voice,[53] *Peter Levine*

These works focus on trauma and how it is experienced by our bodies.

Babette Rothschild specialises in the treatment of trauma and post-traumatic stress disorder, or PTSD – a condition a person may develop after being involved in or witnessing traumatic events such as sexual assault or abuse, warfare, accident or other kinds of threatening situations.

Peter Levine writes on 'Somatic Experiencing®'[54] – a trademarked term to describe his specific approach to working with trauma, which focuses on how we physically process experience in our bodies. He talks about the energy that our body activates in order to deal with some terrifying threat. If it is not used – for instance, if you become overwhelmed and can't move – this energy gets stored up. He writes, "That energy just doesn't go away – it gets locked very deeply in the body. That's the key. It gets locked in the muscles."

It's most easily identified in the war veteran who jumps

at every loud noise. He is constantly scanning all around for danger, his legs are trembling and ready to spring up at any minute, and yet he is sitting in your office, miles and years away from the theatre of war where the trauma happened.

If you think back to a time in your own life when something very frightening happened, you might start to feel those feelings that you felt then, e.g. the tightening in your stomach, your breathing getting shallower, your muscles tensing. You might begin to tremble. It's all still there, often many years after the event. However, it is worth saying here that although many mental health problems stem from traumatic histories, not all do, and traumatic events don't always lead to mental health problems.

People working with other people's trauma often begin to suffer from the effects vicariously. Just listening to and being with great distress, day after day, can take its toll. It's complex work, which requires extensive training, but it can be life changing for people suffering from the long-term effects of trauma. There are courses available, which I found personally helpful after I had read the literature.

6. *THE COURAGE TO HEAL, A GUIDE FOR WOMEN SURVIVORS OF CHILDHOOD SEXUAL ABUSE*[55] BY ELLEN BASS AND LAURA DAVIS

Understanding the legacy of childhood sexual abuse (CSA) is a hugely complex topic. This was the first book that I read on the subject and it was given to me by a woman who had been horribly abused by her father throughout her entire childhood. It is written 'by survivors for survivors'. It was not an easy read and I had to consume it in small doses, taking time and space to digest what I was reading. Many books have since been written on the subject but this one sticks in my mind as having given me a valuable insight into what the effects of CSA might feel like. It also gave me a language to talk about it. It began a dialogue on which I based a lot of my practice. There are many courses available about dealing with CSA.

7. WORKING WITH ADDICTION – *IN THE REALM OF HUNGRY GHOSTS* BY GABOR MATÉ[56]

Working with addiction is difficult for everyone, but for me personally it was probably the hardest area of the work I engaged in. Two of my brothers died fairly young after a life-long struggle with alcohol addiction. It is good to explore your own issues in mental health work. I knew that I found it more difficult to remain positive around issues of addiction and often had to rely on other team members to support me.

The work of Gabor Mate was hugely helpful to me. He works with the most seriously addicted people in the world and talks about his own addictions. The biggest effect his work had on me was to be more compassionate. No one would live the life of addiction by choice. He has worked with hundreds of people affected by addiction and says he has never met someone suffering from addiction who does not have some trauma in their history. The first half of the book contains case histories. So sad were the stories that I got to a point where I felt I could not read on. However, he had made his point; I was feeling much more compassionate and less judgemental when he suddenly switched to the mechanics of addiction, treatment and solutions, which were really helpful and hopeful. His work must have benefited many people. He does lots of online lectures, which are very accessible too.

8. MINDFULNESS AND FOCUSED ATTENTION –
THE POWER OF NOW [57] BY ECKHART TOLL

This book was given to me by one of the volunteers who said it had really helped him. I got to over three quarters of the way through it and felt that I had not really understood it. I was on the point of giving up when it suddenly seemed to be saying something along the lines of, "You might not be getting this yet but just read to the end and you will". It was very spooky – as if he was standing over my shoulder – but it made me carry on. Near the end I suddenly 'got it' and it all made sense to me. The big message to me was to focus on the process not the product. Don't rush to get things finished and thereby lose the experience of the doing.

9. THE APPLICATION OF CONTACT RELATIONS – CARL ROGERS' *A WAY OF BEING*[58] AND GARRY PROUTY'S *PRE-THERAPY*[59]:

Occasionally in a therapeutic garden, we would get a referral for someone from the psychiatric services who was deemed unsuitable for psychiatric intervention or treatment because they were just too unwell to engage with it. Such a person may be out of touch with their own sense of self, other people and their surroundings. They would sometimes appear to be completely lost, bewildered, or even in a kind of dream-like state. The garden sometimes proved to be very therapeutic for people in this condition.

Techniques for working with such a person are explained in Carl Rogers' book *Way of Being*, and also *Pre-therapy: Reaching Contact Impaired Clients* by Garry Prouty, Dion van Werde and Marlis Portner. They talk about allowing people to be their own guide in therapy, and for the people working with them to be congruent, to have unconditional positive regard, and empathy.

All members of the team have to work the same way. The person must not be rushed or expected to do more that they can, and people working with them might need to use a lot of empathic guidance just to help them function safely in the garden.

For example, this person will most likely be unaware of the weather conditions and you might find them out in the garden in very low temperatures and rain without a coat. It might help them to get in touch with their surroundings if you tell them how you feel. This is a very abbreviated version.

> "Goodness, it's really cold today. I'm feeling very cold and I'm wondering if you do too since you don't have a coat on. I think I would really like a hot drink to warm me up. Do you want to come with me to the bothy and get some tea and look for your coat?"

It sounds simplistic but it does seem to work. The person is very out of touch with their feelings, so you have to rely on a bit of guesswork and lend them your own feelings. In this way, people can slowly learn to relate to their surroundings again

10. *RECOVERY: AN ALIEN CONCEPT*[60] BY RON COLEMAN

Ron Coleman is probably one of the earliest speakers and trainers in the recovery/co-production model of mental health work. Along with his wife, Karen Coleman, they have developed an online college which produces many courses and workbooks to support people living with psychosis. Ron is a voice hearer and spent many years in a psychiatric hospital, subjected to every kind of treatment before he "went back to being Ron". He is a charismatic and challenging speaker who talks openly about his own childhood abuse, the traumas that came later in his life, and his eventual experiences of psychosis and hearing voices. I have learnt so much from him.

One of his fundamental beliefs is that recovery cannot happen in isolation. Nor can it happen if the only relationships are based on client and professional interaction. To become whole, you must live and work in society. Becoming whole is not a gift from doctors. It is the responsibility of us all to build that healing society. He is a great believer in people's innate ability to change their own lives.

"If people are the building bricks of recovery then the cornerstone must be self. I believe without reservation that the biggest hurdle we face on our journey to recovery is ourselves. Recovery requires self-confidence, self-esteem, self-awareness and self-acceptance. Without this, recovery is not just impossible, it is not worth it.

We must become confident in our own abilities to change our lives; we must give up being reliant on others doing everything for us. We need to start doing these things for ourselves. We must have the confidence to give up being ill so that we can start being recovered. We must work at raising our self-esteem by becoming citizens within our own communities, despite our communities if need be. We are valued members of our societies and we must recognise our value. We need to recognise our own faults. The system may have created our diagnoses, but often it is ourselves who reinforce it. We need to be aware of our learned behaviour, this should be part of our old lives.

We need to change those behaviours that still trap us in our roles as patients. We need to accept and be proud of who and what we are. I can honestly say my name is Ron Coleman and I am psychotic and proud. This is not a flippant statement, this is a statement of fact." [61]

I was lucky enough to receive some training from Ron and Karen early on in my career and it had a profound influence on the rest of it.

11. TRANSACTIONAL ANALYSIS: *I'M OK, YOU'RE OK* BY THOMAS A HARRIS[62]

"Transactional analysis describes three ego-states (parent, adult and child) as the basis for how we interact and communicate with each other. 'Happy childhood' notwithstanding," says Thomas A Harris. "Most of us are living out the 'Not OK' feelings of a defenceless child wholly dependent on 'OK' others (parents) to look after and care for us. At some stage early in our lives we adopt a 'position' which very significantly determines how we feel about ourselves, particularly in relation to other people. And for a huge portion of the population, that position is 'I'm not OK – You're OK'. This negative 'life position', shared by successful and unsuccessful people alike, contaminates our rational adult potential, leaving us vulnerable to the inappropriate, emotional reactions of our inner child and the uncritically learnt behaviour programmed into our inner parent. By exploring the four basic 'life positions' (I'm ok – you're ok; I'm ok – you're not ok; I'm not ok – you're ok; I'm not ok – you're not ok), we can radically change our lives."

This is a fascinating and enlightening way of looking at relationships and how we get stuck in roles. For example, the twenty-five-year-old 'child' who is a very successful businessman in his own field and has maintained his own home for five years, who comes into his parents' house and reverts to the habitual behaviour of a moody teenager. Or the mother who starts giving advice and instructions to her daughter on the best way to do things, forgetting her daughter is forty years old and a very successful mother of three herself.

The old patterns of behaviour we get stuck in are often responsible for so much misunderstanding. Studying these patterns also helped me develop a much better understanding of the need for small talk and chatting, which I had never been very good at. My husband is very good at it and realises the need for it. It can take him an hour to get along the high street of our small village. He never passes anyone by but will offer a "hello there" to every stranger and a longer chat to anyone who seems to want it. It may sound like small talk, "How are you today", "Nice weather", etc., but what he is really saying is, "I'm OK, you're OK, and we are OK", which offers valuable social cohesion.

Knowing that, because of childhood events, an adult may feel 'not OK' in a very fundamental way even though they appear intelligent, successful, and skilled to the outside world, we can begin to make sense of otherwise confusing behaviour.

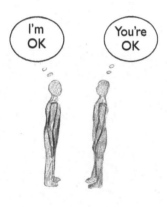

ACKNOWLEDGEMENTS

This book came about after many hours of conversations with my dear friend Catherine Lockerbie, former director of the Edinburgh International Book Festival. After working with me in various gardens and attending training sessions and talks I have given over the years, she pestered me relentlessly to put it all together and write this book. Catherine advised, supported and encouraged me all the way through. Thanks to the kind friends who so generously gave their time to help me. Mary Low and Deirdre MacDonald for photographs, to Joanna Thompson and Robyn Kinsman Blake for their illustrations, which brought the metaphors to life, and to Robert Sless, who helped me with the preparation of the book. He is the most patient IT teacher in the world.

Thanks must also go to my family. To my husband Don, for all the cups of tea and patience he showed while I became obsessed with this project and spent many hours in my office typing away upstairs, and for his total belief that it would happen, and his constant support. He is my rock. (I'm still on the metaphors).

To my two daughters who gave me lots of encouragement and believed I could do it. Although they don't know it, they were many times my solace, light and faith in the future, especially when I came home from work after hearing someone's tragic story which had filled me with sadness. People often used to say they didn't know how I could work full time in a mental health service, with all that it entailed, while bringing up two children. But I truly couldn't have done it without them. Finally, and most important of all, I give my heartfelt thanks to all the people who, over the years, have told me their stories, often at great personal cost. They have shared their wisdom, taught me, worked alongside me and helped me through my own dark days. The great joy and sense of purpose that gardens have given me my whole life long has been enriched by the people I spent time with in them.

Thanks are especially due to two sponsors who have aided in the publication of this book: Reforesting Scotland – Restoring the Land and the People; and Nature Cure in Scotland: Tate Vision Fund, as well as to Fi Martynoga and Madeleine Pollard for their careful editing.

Last but not least, thanks to the following people quoted in this book: Dougie MacLean for permission to reproduce lyrics. 'Scythe Song': Music & Lyrics by Dougie MacLean. Published by Limetree Arts and Music (PRS & MCPS – UK; Kobalt Music/Fintage House – Rest of World). Phil and Poppy Barker for their illuminating teachings (see notes 13, 16, 25, 34 and 35 in References). The inspirational Ron Coleman, quoted from the sources noted in reference notes 60 and 61, and all the authors whose works are cited in the References.

REFERENCES

GROWING WELL IN GARDENS

1. Wilson, Edward O. (1990): *Biophilia*: Harvard University Press.

2. Shinrin-Yoku (forest bathing) – https://www.growwilduk.com/blog/5-simple-steps-practising-shinrin-yoku-forest-bathing

3. Beneficial bacteria in the soil – https://www.permaculture.co.uk/articles/soil-helps-depression

4. Don, Monty. *Gardeners World*, Edition: 31/01/2019, page 17.

5. Community Service Volunteers (now known as Volunteering Matters) – https://volunteering matters.org.uk

6. James Alexander Sinclair.

CHAPTER I

7. Keyes, Corey L. M.: 'The Mental Health Continuum: From Languishing to Flourishing': *Journal of Health and Social Research 2002, Vol. 43* (June): 207–222 (midus.wisc.edu>findings>pdfs>From Languishing to Flourishing).

CHAPTER 2

8. John Muir Trust: Protecting and Managing Wild Land – www.johnmuirtrust.org

CHAPTER 3

9. Levin, Edward D.: Rezvani, Amir H.: 'Nicotinic Interactions with Antipsychotic Drugs, Models of Schizophrenia and Impacts on Cognitive Function': *Biochemical Pharmacology, Vol74, Issue 8, October 2007*: 1182-1191 (www.ncbi.nlm.nih.gov/pmc/articles/PMC2702723/).

CHAPTER 4

10. Levine, Peter (1997): *Walking the Tiger: Healing Trauma – The Innate Capacity to Transform Overwhelming Experiences*: North Atlantic Books; 2016 audiobook: Tantor Media Inc. (www.psychotherapy.net/interview/interview-peter-levine).

CHAPTER 9

11. Don, Monty: Don, Sarah (2005): *The Jewel Garden*: Hodder and Stoughton.

12. A 2007 figure from the Centre for the Economics of Mental Health, quoted in National Mental Health Factfile 3 (can be accessed on www.networks.nhs.uk).

13. Barker, Phil (2004): *The Tidal Model*: Routledge (www.tidal-model.com).

CHAPTER 10

14. Don, Monty. 'How gardening saved my life': *The Observer*, Edition: 9/4/2000.

15. Maté, Gabor. 'In the Realm of Hungry Ghosts': YouTube (www.youtube.com/watch?v=07nOScAHnXI) – 2017 interview, and see note 56 below.

16. *The Tidal Model*, see note 13 above.

17. Depression Alliance – www.depressionalliance.org

18. Johnstone, Mathew (2009): *I Had a Black Dog*: Robinson Publishing (YouTube: 'Living with a black dog', www.youtube.com/watch?v=2VRRx7Mtep8. World health Organisation, WHO).

19. Whitbourne, Susan K. Ph.D. 'How to Deal With Someone Who's Always Looking for a Crisis', Psychology Today, 07/10/2014. (www.psychologytoday.com/gb/blog/fulfillment-any-age/201410/how-deal-someone-whos-always-looking-crisis), page 96.

REFERENCES

CHAPTER 11

20. Panic Attacks: for information:
www.lifeline.org.au/get-help/topics/panic-attacks

21. Anxiety: www.supportline.org.uk/problems/anxiety

CHAPTER 12

22. Briggs, Raymond (1980): *The Snowman*: Puffin.

23. John Muir Trust, *see above*.

24. Edwin Morgan (2002): 'At Eighty', from *Cathures: New Poems 1990–2001*, Carcanet.

25. *The Tidal Model*, see note 13 above.

CHAPTER 13

26. 'Scythe Song', Dougie MacLean (see Acknowledgements).

27. Homer, *Iliad*.

28. Buzan, Tony (1995): *The Mind Map Book*: BBC Consumer Publishing.

29. Waite, Terry: Coles, Jenny (2016): *Out of the Silence: Memories, Poems, Reflections*: SPCK Publishing, and Waite, Terry (1993): *Taken On Trust* (kindle): Harcourt.

30. Solution Focused Therapy, Counselling Directory www.counselling-directory.org.uk/solution-focused-brief-therapy.html

31. Metcalf, Linda (2006): *The Miracle Question: Answer It and Change Your Life*: Crown House Publishing.

CHAPTER 14

32. Griffin, Joe; Tyrell, Ivan (2004: *Human Givens*: HG Publishing (Human Givens Institute: www.hgi.org.uk).

33. *Human Givens*, see above.

34. *The Tidal Model*, see note 13 above.

35. The Tidal Metaphor, on www.tidal-model.com

36. Keyes, Corey: see note 7 above.

37. Return to Now: 'Why Aborigines Don't Have Words for "Please" or "Thank You"'. (https://returntonow. net/2017/01/26/aborigines-dont-say-please-or-thank-you/).

38. Pinkerton, Susan (2015): *The Village Effect, Why Face to Face Contact Matters*: Atlantic Books, page 215.

39. McCulloch, Janet M.D.: Ramesar, Simon: Peterson, Heather: 'Psychotherapy in Primary Care: The BATHE Technique': *American Family Physician.* May 1998. 1;57(9): 2131-2134. (www.aafp.org/afp/1998/0501/p2131.html).

40. Jeffers, Susan (2007): *Feel The Fear and Do It Anyway*: Vermilion.

41. Moodgym: online self-help for depression and anxiety – https://moodgym.com.au/

42. Johnson, Spencer (1999) *Who Moved my Cheese?* Vermilion, paperback ed.

43. *I Had a Black Dog*, see note 18 above.

44. Graham, Linda. 'The Triangle Of Victim, Rescuer, Persecutor – What It Is and How To Get Out'. https://lindagraham-mft. net/triangle-victim-rescuer-persecutor-get/

45. Deikman, Arthur, J. (1983): *The Observing Self: Mysticism and Psychotherapy*: Beacon Press.

CHAPTER 15

46.Rosenberg, Marshall B. (2015): *Nonviolent Communication: A Language of Life*: Puddle Dancer Press. Rosenberg, Marshall B. (2005): *The Surprising Purpose of Anger*: Puddle Dancer Press. (www.compassionatecommunication.co.uk-non-violent communication/NVC).

47. AVP: Alternatives To Violence – https://avpbritain.org.uk

48. Alexander, F.M. (2018):*The Use of Self*: Orion (https://alexan-

REFERENCES

dertechnique.co.uk/alexander-technique).

49. Suicide prevention training:
https://www.prevent-suicide.org.uk

50. Rothschild, Babette (2000): *The Body Remembers*: Norton and Company.

51. Rothschild, Babette (2006): *Help for the Helper*: Norton and Company.

52. Levine, Peter (1997): *Walking the Tiger: Healing Trauma-The Innate Capacity to Transform Overwhelming Experiences*: North Atlantic Books.

53. Levine, Peter (2010), *In an Unspoken Voice: How the Body Releases Trauma and Restores Goodness:* North Atlantic Books.

54. Somatic Experiencing®: https://traumahealing.org

55. Bass, Ellen: Davis, Laura:(2002*): The Courage to Heal: A Guide for Women Survivors of Childhood Sexual Abuse:* Vermilion.

56. Maté, Gabor (2018): *In the Realm of Hungry Ghosts: Close Encounters with Addiction*: Vermilion.

57. Tolle, Eckhart (2016): *The Power of Now*: Yellow Kite.

58. Rogers, Carl (1980): *A Way of Being*: Mariner Books.

59. Prouty, Garry et al (2002): *Pre-therapy: Reaching Contact Impaired Clients*: PCCS Books.

60. Coleman, Ron (2018): *Recovery: An Alien Concept*: Create Space Independent Publishing Platform.

61. Ron Coleman, quoted from: https://www.scottishrecovery.net/resource/stepping-stones-to-recovery/

OTHER USEFUL BOOKS AND WEBSITES
In recent years, there has been a huge growth in the number of books and websites about mental health and eco-therapy, both professional and popular. Below is a list of some others that strongly influenced my thinking and the approaches discussed throughout this book.

Husvedt, Siri (2010): *The Shaking Woman or a History of My Nerves*: Spectre

Rowe, Dorothy (2003): *Depression: The Way Out of Your Prison*: Routledge

Keen, Sam (1992): *Fire in the Belly: On Being a Man*: Bantam USA

Van Der Kolk, Bessel (2015): *The Body Keeps the Score: Mind, Brain and Body Transformation*: Penguin

Rogers, Carl (1995): *A Way of Being*: Mariner Books

Sutton, Jan (2007): *Healing the Hurt Within, Understanding Self-injury and Self-harm, and Heal the Emotional Wounds*: How To Books

Servan-Shreiber, David (2012): *Healing Without Freud or Prozac*: Rodale

www.hearing-voicesnetwork.org.uk

www.workingtorecovery.co.uk

www.samaritans.org

www.farmgarden.org.uk

www.thrive.org.uk

www.trellisscotland.org.uk

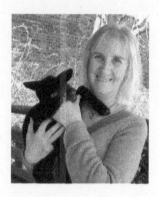

Jan Cameron has worked in community gardens and therapeutic environments for forty years and has seen first-hand in many different contexts how gardening directly benefits our health. She has spent three years as a youth worker, ten years working in a residential school for distressed children, twenty-five years in mental health training gardens and six years working in community gardens – as well as training people in the principles and practice of therapeutic horticulture. She has delivered training for Thrive, Trellis, TCV, Community Farm Gardens, Scottish Recovery Network, Depression Alliance and the Scottish Association for Mental Health. She holds qualifications in fields including social work, as a Practice Educator, in suicide prevention (ASSIST), and horticulture training. She lives in the Scottish Borders, and this is her first book.